Professionalism in Tomorrow's Healthcare System

Towards Fulfilling the ACGME Requirements for Systems-Based Practice and Professionalism

Professionalism in Tomorrow's Healthcare System

Towards Fulfilling the ACGME Requirements for Systems-Based Practice and Professionalism

Edited by
Ann E. Mills, Donna T. Chen,
Patricia H. Werhane,
and Matthew K. Wynia

Hagerstown 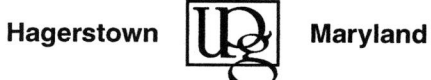 Maryland

University Publishing Group, Inc.
Hagerstown, Maryland 21740
1(800)654-8188
www.UPGBooks.com
Copyright © 2005 by University Publishing Group
All rights reserved
Printed in the United States of America

ISBN 1-55572-037-4

No part of this publication may be reproduced, stored in a retrieval system, or transmitted, in any form, or by any means, electronic, mechanical, photocopying, recording or otherwise, without the prior written permission of University Publishing Group.

The artwork on the cover is fractal of the day for 21 June 1996, created by Julien Clinton Sprott, PhD, Professor of Physics, University of Wisconsin, Madison, *http://sprott.physics.wisc.edu*. © 2005 Julien Clinton Sprott, used with permission, all rights reserved.

Earlier versions of chapters 1, 3, 4, 6, 7, and 11 first appeared in *Organizational Ethics: Healthcare, Business, and Policy*, 2, no. 1 (Spring 2005). © 2005 University Publishing Group, used with permission, all rights reserved.

The tables in chapter 5 are adapted from material first published in J.D. Voss, M.M. Nadkarni, and J.M. Schectman, "The Clinical Health Economics System Simulation," *Academic Medicine* 80, no. 2 (February 2005): 129-34, lists 1 and 2, and table 2. © 2005, Lippincott Williams & Wilkins, used with permission, all rights reserved.

The ACGME General Competencies in the appendix are used with the permission of the Accreditation Council for Graduate Medical Education. © ACGME 2005, all rights reserved.

Contents

Introduction   vii
Ann E. Mills, Donna T. Chen, Patricia H. Werhane, and Matthew K. Wynia

Professionalism

1. Towards a New Concept of Professionalism: Being a Physician in Today's Healthcare System   3
   Edward M. Spencer and Rebecca Bigoney

2. Towards Systems-Informed Professionalism   21
   Donna T. Chen, Ann E. Mills, and Patricia H. Werhane

3. The Ethical Climate: Can Organizational Ethics Programs Influence Management Initiatives?   43
   Paul A. Clark

The Financial Perspective

4. Professionalism in Medicine and in Business   67
   Lisa H. Newton

5. The Clinical Health Economics System Simulation (CHESS): A New Tool for Promoting Competency in Systems-Based Practice and Professionalism   83
   John D. Voss, Natalie B. May, and Joel M. Schectman

Internal Patient Care and Business Processes

6. Business Practices, Ethical Principles, and Professionalism   101
   Ann E. Mills and Mary V. Rorty

7. Individuals, Systems, and Professional Behavior   125
   Evan G. DeRenzo

Learning and Growth

8. Professionalism, Humanism, Mindfulness, and the Healthcare Melee   151
   Daniel M. Becker and Matthew J. Goodman

The Patient's Perspective

9. Through the Looking Glass: The Patient's Point of View   169
   Daniel M. Becker

Residency Training and Outcomes Assessment

10. Educating for Systems-Informed Professionalism   181
    Donna T. Chen and Ann E. Mills

11. The Challenges of a Residency Education Program for Competencies in Organizational Ethics   209
    David T. Ozar

12. The Patient's Perspective in the ACGME Systems-Based Competency   227
    Walter S. Davis

13. Training Residents for Excellence in Systems-Based Clinical Practices: Management of Blood Draws as the Quintessential Outcome Measure   239
    Evan G. DeRenzo, Phil Buescher, and Kirsten Alcorn

    Summary and Conclusion   253
    Ann E. Mills, Donna T. Chen, Patricia H. Werhane, and Matthew K. Wynia

    Appendix: The ACGME Outcome Project General Competencies   265

    Contributors   269

    Index   273

Introduction

*Ann E. Mills, Donna T. Chen,
Patricia H. Werhane, and Matthew K. Wynia*

We address this book to medical educators, physicians, administrators, and residents who are interested in the appropriate development and implementation of the Accreditation Council for Graduate Medical Education (ACGME) competencies on systems-based practice and professionalism.

REFORMING RESIDENT EDUCATION

The Outcome Project was initiated by the ACGME to train physicians to deal with the complexities of a changing healthcare environment.[1] It was launched in 1999 with the identification of six general areas of expertise or "core competencies" that residency training programs should teach and monitor:

- Patient care,
- Medical knowledge,
- Practice-based learning and improvement,
- Interpersonal and communication skills,
- Professionalism, and
- System-based practice.

The full text of the ACGME General Competencies is included as an appendix in this volume.

These competencies were fleshed out during the second phase of the Outcome Project, which ended in 2002. The third phase, projected to end in 2006, is intended to sharpen the focus of the competencies and the assessment tools designed to measure them. Later phases will focus on integrating the competencies into residency training and assessing educational outcomes. Although the Outcome Project is directed toward residency training, it will likely generalize to undergraduate medical education and to the certification and recertification processes of practicing physicians. Thus, it is expected to influence the whole continuum of medical education and professional development.[2]

The Outcome Project focuses on both content and assessment. It details the expertise and obligations required in each of the six areas. It directs the attention of medical educators to measuring the outcomes associated with the educational programs. The ACGME website offers resources for those responsible for implementing the competencies.[3] Under each competency are references and examples of possible ways of implementing the educational and assessment tools. The focus on outcomes is an attempt to overcome the failures associated with merely focusing on controlling processes, failures that have been seen elsewhere in the healthcare delivery system.[4]

Academic health centers are currently scrambling to understand and implement the competencies. Since the ACGME leaves the specifics of implementation and measurement to the individual residency programs, so far there is no benchmark or "best practice" that individual programs can measure their results against. This is expected to change when the project begins its fourth phase in 2011, when more data presumably will be available. But for now there is considerable ambiguity about the content defined in the competencies, their implementation in residency programs, and the appropriateness of various assessment tools.

BUSINESS PRACTICES AND THE ROLE OF ETHICS IN THE HEALTHCARE SYSTEM

The ACGME competency on systems-based practice requires that "residents . . . demonstrate an awareness of and responsiveness to the larger context and system of health care." This competency emphasizes the interrelationship of the different elements and levels of the healthcare system. It calls attention to the importance of position and role in the system as determinants of responsibilities, urges consideration of cost control and resource allocation, and points out the responsibility of the physician as educator of and advocate for the patient within the larger system.

The Outcome Project thus specifies, at the level of resident education, a systems-thinking approach that has characterized recent reports by the Institute of Medicine (IOM). The 2000 IOM report, *Crossing the Quality Chasm,* takes a systems-based approach to quality improvement in the healthcare system at all levels, and highlights, in the course of its lengthy investigation, the extent to which decisions and procedures at any level affect and are affected by decisions and procedures at all other levels.[5] According to the IOM, our present healthcare system is a complex "adaptive system," which is defined as "a complex of [evolving] interacting components together with the networks of relationships among them that identify an entity and/or a set of processes."[6] According to Susan Wolf, who has studied systems of managed care, "a truly systemic view [of healthcare] considers how a set of individuals, institutions and processes operates in a system involving a complex network of interrelationships, an array of individual and institutional actors with conflicting interests and goals, and a number of feedback loops."[7]

The introduction of the competency on systems-based practice for residents recognizes the importance of this insight, as well as the central role the physician plays in the healthcare system as a whole. Understanding of the larger system and the interdependence of its components among physicians is crucial to the development and maintenance of a healthcare system in the United States that will meet the needs of its citizenry in a professionally responsible manner.

The ACGME competency addressing professionalism adds to the responsibility of the medical professional the need to "demonstrate . . . a commitment to ethical principles pertaining to . . . *business practices"* (emphasis is ours). Taken together, these two competencies move professionalism from its traditional focus on the individual physician to focus on how the individual physician interacts with, and is influenced by and through, the systems that deliver and finance healthcare. Moreover, these two competencies require that the physician, as a professional, assume some responsibility for the appropriate functioning of the systems delivering care and the values these systems reflect.

These requirements echo and reinforce the introduction, in 1995, by the Joint Commission on Accreditation of Healthcare Organizations (JCAHO), of a requirement for accreditation that requires healthcare organizations to conduct their business practices in an "honest, decent and proper manner," in light of the primacy of the value of patient care.[8] Scholars and practitioners responding to this focus are working in an area that JCAHO called "organization ethics."[9] Organization ethics (or "organizational ethics") focuses on organizations, the mezzo level of the healthcare system, between individual clinical encounters and systemic features of care, and considers how business practices affect the healthcare organization, its stakeholders, and its ability to provide healthcare. Seated as it is in the middle, organizational ethics thus expands the range of considerations appropriate for an ethical evaluation of healthcare processes beyond the conventional focus on the individual physician-patient interaction, a micro level system. In healthcare, organizational ethics can acknowledge the ethical primacy of that physician-patient relationship, while also drawing into consideration the roles of other stakeholders whose decisions, constraints, and interactions have an impact upon decision making. In effect, the JCAHO mandate is a requirement that the patient care and business practices associated with healthcare delivery integrate the values of individual, organizational, and systemic ethics.

As is appropriate for its role as accreditor of hospitals, medical centers, and other healthcare organizations, the JCAHO mandate focuses on the organizational level. By including the requirement to "demonstrate . . . a commitment to ethical principles pertaining to . . . *business practices,*" the ACGME also suggests that physicians' professionalism should include the values associated with traditional medical ethics *and* business ethics. Healthcare organizations, of course, are systems embedded in a larger nationwide (and even more broadly, global) macro healthcare system. What we can learn from organizational ethics is thus important to thinking across all levels of the healthcare system.

SYSTEMS-BASED PRACTICE, ORGANIZATIONAL ETHICS, AND THE ETHICAL CLIMATE

When the Outcome Project was initiated in 1999, persons interested in organizational ethics were still formulating their

Introduction

ideas about what organizational ethics could mean for healthcare, healthcare institutions, and individual healthcare professionals. Nevertheless, what has emerged promises to be very useful in sharpening the focus of the ACGME competencies, particularly the competencies in professionalism and systems-based practice.

Organizational ethics for healthcare focuses on *healthcare organizations.* It is concerned that healthcare organizations conduct their business practices in an "honest, decent and proper manner," keeping in mind the primacy of the value of patient care. Organizational ethics is concerned with how the values espoused by the organization are reflected in the activities of the organization — its systems, processes, and procedures, and the policies that surround the delivery of care. It is concerned with the beliefs and behaviors of individual or groups of organization stakeholders and whether or not these beliefs and behaviors are aligned with the values of the organization. In short, the concern of organizational ethics is with the ethical climate of the organization — and the goal of healthcare organizational ethics is to articulate and maintain a positive ethical climate in the healthcare organization. (The "organizational ethical climate" consists of the shared perceptions of the "general and pervasive characteristics of [an] organization [of a system] affecting a broad range of decisions.")[10]

A positive ethical climate has at least two important characteristics. First, it is an organizational culture in which the mission and vision of the organization inform the expectations for professional and managerial performance and are implemented in the actual practices of the organization. Second, a positive ethical climate embodies a set of values that reflect societal norms for what the organization should value, how it should prioritize is mission, vision, and goals, and how the organization and the individuals associated with it should behave.

The ACGME competency on "professionalism" deals with some of the traditional concepts of medical ethics and clinical ethics, like informed consent and confidentiality, but it also obliges physicians to commit to the "ethical principles pertaining to . . . business practices." By doing so, the ACGME asks physicians to widen their perspectives to consider the content and consequences of their decisions and actions from the perspective of business practices and the principals that underline them. It suggests that physicians have some level of responsibility for the ethical climate of the healthcare organizations in which they function, and even, by implication, for the functioning of the macro healthcare system.

While it is still a new field, healthcare organizational ethics directs attention to how the mission of the organization — to provide excellent care at reasonable cost — is carried out throughout the organization in its business and patient care practices, and works to bring its relationships, processes, procedures, and policies — at all levels of function — in line with its mission of excellent patient care. This approach is directly related to the competency on systems-based practice, because all systems *are constituted by* relationships, processes, procedures, and policies. What one's roles and responsibilities are in a particular system are defined by that system. And because systems determine the environment in which people work, systems influence their beliefs and behaviors, which affects the ethical climate of the organization. But the ethical climate of any organization or larger system will also affect decision making, which in turn will influence the way systems evolve. Thus, there is a two-way relationship between the activities of any organization and its ethical climate — each affects the other. Similarly, there is a two-way relationship between the roles, responsibilities, and activities of physicians working in systems-based practices and their sense of professional identity and integrity — their professionalism.

Organizations and organizational ethics provide a context to explore these competencies on professionalism and systems-based practice. But even if we concede that these two competencies should be explored within this context, we are still left with a number of questions. What does the inclusion of a competency that requires physicians to commit to the ethical principles pertaining to business practices *mean* in terms of the traditional concept of medical professionalism? The goal of business practices is to produce care of optimal value, which also implies cost-effective care. Can our traditional understanding of professionalism be reconciled with such an obligation? What are the important characteristics of business practices? Are they the same across all healthcare organizations, or should they be? How can they support or impede professionalism? Can a system reconcile the competing objectives of its component levels and units? What does it mean for residents to learn to work within a system? What

Introduction

kind of education is required for residents in this regard? How can it be developed? How can it be taught and assessed?

This book addresses these issues though four primary objectives. The first objective is to investigate some of the questions raised by the introduction of competencies on systems-based practice and professionalism that include the ethics of business practices. The second objective is to explore these competencies within the context of organizational ethics. The third objective is to suggest a way that residents can organize this wider perspective, which they must acquire to meet the requirements of the competencies. And the fourth objective is to discuss how the competencies can be taught and assessed.

To meet these objectives, we have gathered a group composed of scholars, medical and resident educators, ethicists, administrators, and practicing physicians. We have asked them what these two competencies might mean for physicians and residents in their practice and their education. We have asked them to explore the interconnections as well as the limitations of organizational ethics in addressing the two competencies. We have asked them to consider what "systems" thinking might mean and what professionalism might mean in the context of a system, and how it might be taught.

•   •   •

Physicians are defined by their professionalism and the values associated with it. Without these values, physicians can be viewed as technicians, albeit highly skilled technicians. Because professionalism is so embedded in physicians' identities, we start with questions of what the introduction of ACGME competencies on systems-based practice and professionalism (which includes a commitment to ethical principles associated with business practices) might mean to our traditional understanding of professionalism, and whether or not professionalism can be expanded to include a systems perspective.

The chapter, "Toward a New Concept of Professionalism: Being a Physician in Today's Healthcare System," by Edward M. Spencer and Rebecca Bigoney, examines more closely the concept of professionalism in medicine. The authors argue that the inclusion of a "commitment to the ethical principles pertaining to provision or withholding of clinical care, confidentiality of patient information, informed consent, and business practices," along with the goal of the systems-based practice competency, "to deliver care of optimal value," requires that the physician's moral vision must widen to include issues not traditionally considered to be relevant to the physician's professionalism. But, they ask, will this be efficient or effective within the context of the wider system, where some interactions cannot be controlled? They point out the limitations of organizational ethics, as it has developed in this context, and argue that the combination of the two ACGME competencies means that the physician has a role in ensuring the successful functioning of the system as a whole. But, they claim, this role has not been properly defined, either by the competencies or by professional associations. They conclude by discussing some responses by physicians and the "system" that can possibly assure that a somewhat different, but nevertheless legitimate, moral landscape for the practicing physician can be developed and maintained, so that all stakeholders can continue to understand what it means to be a physician in a moral sense.

In the essay that follows, "Towards Systems-Informed Professionalism," Donna T. Chen, Ann E. Mills, and Patricia H. Werhane begin thinking about what professionalism might mean in the context of "systems." They begin by describing a system and its characteristics — its purpose, its processes, the resources required, and its survival needs. They link these characteristics to the elements of a strategic management tool, the Balanced Scorecard, developed by Robert Kaplan and David Norton out of concern that businesses were not being appropriately managed for success in an increasingly competitive world, who argued that any organization that wanted to survive for the long-term needed to pay attention to (1) the perspective of the customer, (2) its internal processes, (3) the needs of persons associated with the organization, and (4) the financial needs of the organization.[11]

Because the components of the Balanced Scorecard can, with only minor modifications, correspond to the characteristics of any human system, Chen, Mills, and Werhane use it as their starting point and discuss how a resident can acquire a "systems-informed" perspective. But they argue that such a framework will not point physicians toward the "right" answers or "correct" decisions. For that, physicians will need the goals and the values, and their prioritization, that is supplied by professional-

Introduction

ism, thus moving a systems-informed perspective to a perspective that is characterized by what might be called a "systems-informed professionalism." Chen, Mills, and Werhane show how systems-informed professionalism integrates the expectations of the ACGME competencies on professionalism and systems-based practice — and, indeed, how systems-informed professionalism encompasses all of the ACGME competencies.

The authors point out that, in the same way organizations can modify the framework supplied by the Balanced Scorecard to suit their specific needs and objectives, resident educators can modify systems-informed professionalism to the realities of their own institutions. But, they argue, if the delivery of quality cost-effective care is the goal of the competencies, then a systems perspective is required to help balance competing needs. Their chapter suggests one way of developing this perspective.

Paul A. Clark's essay, "The Ethical Climate: Can Organizational Ethics Programs Influence Management Initiatives?" is not directed at the competencies or resident education. It is directed to organizational ethicists as they struggle to find ways to influence organizational decision making. The language used and the issues addressed are not commonly associated with resident education, but we include this chapter to discuss some of the complexities that are associated with organizational decision making, and to show how organizations can design systems so that competing obligations *can* be balanced in decision making, and outcomes be measured. Moreover, as we have said, the competencies require attention to the values that are associated with traditional medical ethics and the ethical principals pertaining to business practices. Clark uses the Balanced Scorecard to illustrate how these values and principals are important in the formation of any business practice that is associated with healthcare. Thus, Clark provides us with an example of how systems thinking can be used at the organization level to achieved desired outcomes.

Taken together, these three chapters address issues associated with traditional medical ethics and business practices at every level in the delivery system.

Because we can make a correlation between systems and the components of the Balanced Scorecard, we have a framework with which to explore the tensions, the conceptual difficulties, and the interconnections of the two ACGME competencies, the delivery system, and organizational ethics. Thus, the sections that follow correlate to the framework supplied by the Balanced Scorecard. We begin with the financial perspective, because fiscal solvency represents the minimal effectiveness needed for a human system, like a healthcare organization, to survive. We are not suggesting that the financial perspective should be dominant; we merely use this label to explore the tensions within the delivery system.

This section begins with Lisa H. Newton's essay on the differing concepts of professionalism associated with medicine and business. In her chapter, "Professionalism in Medicine and in Business," Newton describes the changing healthcare system, the challenges that physicians face, and the anomalies the system has produced. She discusses the conflicting fiduciary obligations of physicians and managers — and asks whether or not these obligations can be resolved. This essay highlights the difficulties and conflicts that physicians face when their decision making occurs in the context of scare resources. It is readable and lively, and might serve the resident educator well in introducing the healthcare system and the constraints it imposes on the physician.

The essay by John D. Voss, Natalie B. May, and Joel M. Schectman, "The Clinical Health Economics System Simulation (CHESS): A New Tool for Promoting Competency in Systems-based Practice and Professionalism," directly confronts the financial issues raised by the competencies. Voss, May, and Schectman introduce a computer model that is used to heighten residents' awareness of what cost-effectiveness might mean in the delivery of care, and provides concrete examples that lead to discussions of the ethical issues that are embedded in financial decision making.

The next section, on patient care and business practices, addresses roles and responsibilities: the relationships, systems, processes, procedures, and policies that surround the delivery of care. It is composed of two essays. Ann E. Mills and Mary V. Rorty address questions of what business practices are and why business processes may fail to produce desired outcomes in chapter six, "Business Practices, Ethical Principles, and Professionalism." They begin by noting that business practices have normative content. They look at some characteristics of business practices and speculate that, as has sometimes been true in the past, the pressures of business considerations might invite other

Introduction

organizations in the delivery system to seek ways of undermining traditional medical professionalism. They conclude that enlarging the concept of professionalism to include greater consideration of cost will not be enough for physicians and the organizations with which they are affiliated to achieve the goals of the competencies on professionalism and systems-based practice. Doing so will demand that the system, as a whole, commit to the same goals. This essay does not ignore the importance of a positive organizational ethical climate as a necessary condition for excellence in physician practice. On the contrary, the fact that business processes have normative content invites scrutiny from organizational ethics programs and those associated with them. Organizational ethics programs might also help in the identification and articulation of physicians' roles if their moral vision must be widened as demanded by the competencies.

In the next essay, Evan G. DeRenzo returns the focus on how the organization and the systems it uses affect the individual. DeRenzo's essay, "Individuals, Systems, and Professional Behavior," focuses on the systems that make up the patient care practices of a healthcare organization. She points out that mastering scientific and clinical knowledge, the core skills of the medically competent physician, are not the skills considered primary for mastery of systems-based practice. Competency in a systems-based practice will require a different set of skills, specifically the mastery of complex psychological responses and the ability to engage in refined yet vigorous ethical debate.

DeRenzo uses a series of case examples to illustrate that developing these skills in residents will require a morally safe environment. But a morally safe environment is an environment that reflects a positive ethical climate, which, as we have discussed, is the province of organizational ethics.

The competency on systems-based practice requires that physicians work to improve the system in which they practice. Rather than focus on various skills that physicians must acquire as they practice, in the next section, "Learning and Growth," we have chosen to include a more personal essay written by two physicians in practice, in part as a reminder that, regardless of the systems level focus, it is individuals who make up these systems, and it is individuals who are affected by these systems.

In their essay, "Professionalism, Humanism, Mindfulness, and the Healthcare Melee," Daniel M. Becker and Matthew J. Goodman illustrate their frustrations with the delivery system.

They demonstrate how their focus on producing desirable outcomes with and for patients is disrupted because of the various systems within which they interact. Becker and Goodman turn to "mindfulness" as a way to regain their focus and remind themselves why they are physicians.

"Mindfulness" is the ability to disengage from a conflict or dilemma without passion or prejudice And, although Becker and Goodman's focus is on using "mindfulness" to relieve stress, to regain the calm and composure that physicians need as they carry out their daily tasks, it serves another purpose. The ability to disengage from a dilemma or conflict also allows physicians to reflect on the nature of a problem with a view to reaching some sort of resolution: it allows the deployment of what Patricia Werhane has called "moral imagination."[12]

Essays in this book have used what might be considered by physicians to be novel terminology and concepts. Various essays have focused on "systems," on "organizational climate," on "conflicts," on "barriers to achieving desired outcomes." Nevertheless, as Donald Berwick, one of the architects of the IOM report *Crossing the Quality Chasm* points out, the quality of actions at any level of the healthcare delivery system "ought to be defined as the effects of those actions . . . on the experience of patients, their loved ones, and the communities in which they live."[13] Thus, lest we forget *why* we are addressing these systems issues, we have asked Daniel M. Becker to write a personal essay describing the "patient's perspective."

In this essay, Becker describes a case in which the patient and physician have a long-term relationship. Becker describes how this relationship unfolds within the context of the delivery system. We see what "optimal" care might mean to both patient and physician, and we see what outcomes are eventually produced. We also see the costs of these outcomes to both the physician and patient, and the costs are by no means only financial in nature. And we realize that part of the problem is that both of these individuals seem to have little control over the systems that seek to influence their decision making.

Our next section is concerned with residency training and outcomes assessment. Each essay focuses on a separate aspect of what will be entailed in educating residents in systems-based practice and in a professionalism that includes a commitment to the ethical principles of business practices. But, even though the essays are diverse, there are numerous connections.

Introduction

Donna T. Chen and Ann E. Mills, in "Educating for Systems-Informed Professionalism," build on chapter two, in which Chen, Mills, and Werhane argue that a systems perspective is necessary to achieve the requirements of the competency on systems-based practice, but that decision making must take place within the parameters supplied by the values associated with professionalism. In chapter two, Chen, Mills, and Werhane developed a framework that they called "systems-informed professionalism," and showed how this framework integrates the expectations of the competencies on professionalism and systems-based practice — and, indeed, may encompass all of the ACGME competencies. In this chapter, Chen and Mills outline the skills, knowledge, and sensitivities that promote systems-informed professionalism, and show how they can be incorporated into the medical education and professional development process. They are careful to point out that systems-informed professionalism requires the ability to (1) disengage or to use mindfulness to put a space between the physician and the situation at hand, and (2) that only by being mindful can a physician begin to use moral imagination — part of the moral reasoning process.

David T. Ozar, in his chapter, "The Challenges of a Residency Education Program for Competencies in Organizational Ethics," discusses a curricular approach to developing the knowledge, skills, and sensitivities required by moral reasoning in the context of organizational or system practice. Ozar also sees in the ACGME competencies that physicians should take a leadership role and work to improve the systems in which they practice. And, he suggests the specific skills necessary to achieve this — both on the part of the educator, and for the physicians of the future.

Walter S. Davis looks at the patient's perspective in the ACGME competency on systems-based practice, a key element of professionalism in systems-based practice. He explores how the patient's perspective can be incorporated into educating and evaluating residents in systems-based practice.

Finally, Evan G. DeRenzo, Phil Buescher, and Kirsten Alcorn, in their chapter, "Training Residents for Excellence in System-Based Clinical Practices: Management of Blood Draws as the Quintessential Outcome Measure," argue that clinically appropriate management of blood draws in the critical care setting could serve as an educational outcome measure that would incorporate not just the competencies on professionalism and systems-based practice, but all of the ACGME competencies They argue that focusing attention on this is one way to educate residents about clinically and ethically appropriate management of blood products throughout the healthcare delivery system. It is a good example of one of the ways in which small, routine decisions afford opportunities to address the ACGME competencies in a way that is relevant to practice.

•   •   •

The ACGME has an ambitious agenda, and, despite the confusions that attend it in these initial stages, all indications are that it is an agenda with a positive future. It acknowledges and integrates insights worked out on other levels of the healthcare system, and urges that they be incorporated in residency education. Residents will be trained with an eye towards these competencies — and educational programs will be assessed as to how well they have achieved their goals. But more is at stake than the revision of resident education. Residents are tomorrow's physicians; they are, as many managed-care companies have discovered, at the core of the delivery system. They are the gateway to the costs of the system, and they are central to its success in terms of a professionalism that has, until recently, been defined primarily in terms of the physician-patient relationship. The ACGME Outcome Project acknowledges the extent to which this is changing. It suggests that physicians have the obligation to commit to the ethical principles of business practices with the goal of delivering quality cost-effective care.

Business practices and patient care practices constitute healthcare systems, and each can operate on the micro, mezzo, and macro levels. Residents and other physicians practice within a healthcare system that includes physicians, many other stakeholders, and healthcare organizations. Organizations and systems influence and guide decision making for those within them, and, as a result, in healthcare, "the system" will often have direct effects on health outcomes. So physicians who are devoted to patient care can no longer, if they ever could, divorce themselves from the consequences of the ways in which systems are designed, the goals they seek to achieve, and the outcomes they produce. To help improve these systems, physicians are being asked to develop an understanding of the characteristics of organizations and systems, and how to mold them.

We invite the comments of our colleagues in medical education and professional development across the spectrum as we struggle to prepare the next generation of physicians in a healthcare system that is in transition. We do not pretend to answer some of the larger questions raised by the essays. Nor do we pretend to have addressed all of the questions raised by the competencies on systems-based practice and professionalism. These questions include the formation and adoption of a goal and the values that drive it for *all* of the components of the delivery system, and how best to align them with an organizational ethic that will be reflected in the more micro systems of clinical practice. In the meantime, raising the systemic issues of competing obligations on the mezzo level of the healthcare organization and the micro level of clinical practice may help the physicians of the future come to these discussions with a better idea of what their role *should* be in the successful functioning of the delivery system, and how to reconcile that role with the traditional medical ethics perspective that has been the time-honored commitment of professionals.

NOTES

1. ACGME Outcome Project, *http://www.acgme.org/outcome/comp/compFull.asp.*
2. C. Carroccio et al., "Educating the Pediatrician of the 21st Century: Defining and Implementing a Competency Based System," *Pediatrics* 113, no. 2 (February 2004): 252-8.
3. See note 1 above.
4. J.C. Robinson, "The end of managed care," *Journal of the American Medical Association* 285, no. 20 (2001): 2622-8.
5. Institute of Medicine, Committee on Quality and Health Care in America, *Crossing the Quality Chasm: A New Health System for the 21st Century* (Washington D.C.: National Academy Press, 2001). Of particular relevance is the appendix by Paul Plsek, "Redesigning health care with insights from the science of complex adaptive systems," pp. 310-333.
6. A. Laszlo and S. Krippner, "Systems Theories: Their Origins, Foundations and Development," in *Systems Theories and a Priori Aspects of Perception,* ed. J.S. Jordan (Amsterdam: Elsevier, 1988), 47-74.
7. S. Wolf, "Toward a Systemic Theory of Informed Consent in Managed Care," *Houston Law Review* 35 (1999): 1631-81.

8. Joint Commission on Accreditation on Healthcare Organizations, "Patient Rights and Organizational Ethics: Standards for Organizational Ethics," *Comprehensive Manual for Hospitals* (Oakbrook Terrace Ill.: Joint Commission on Accreditation on Healthcare Organizations, 1996), 95-7.

9. In the fall of 1999, *The Journal of Clinical Ethics* published a special issue on Organizational Ethics, edited by Robert Potter, volume 10, no. 3 (Fall 1999). Almost simultaneously *HEC Forum* published a special issue on Organization Ethics, volume 8, no. 4 (1999). Several books were published, including E.M. Spencer et al., *Organization Ethics in Health Care* (New York: Oxford University Press, 2000) and K.L. Wong, *Medicine and the Marketplace* (Notre Dame, Ind.: University of Notre Dame Press, 1998). See also D. Ozar et al., *Organization Ethics in Health Care: Toward a Model for Ethical Decision Making by Provider Organizations*, a report by the American Medical Association Institute of Ethics National Working Group (Chicago, Ill.: AMA, 2001), 17.

10. B. Victor and J. Cullen, "The Organizational Bases of Ethical Work Climates," *Administrative Science Quarterly* 33, (1988): 101-25.

11. R.S. Kaplan and D.P. Norton, *The Balanced Scorecard: Translating Strategy into Action* (Boston, Mass.: Harvard Business School Press, 1996).

12. P.H. Werhane, *Moral Imagination and Management Decision Making* (New York: Oxford University Press, 1999).

13. D.M. Berwick, "A user's manual for the IOM's 'Quality Chasm' report," *Health Affairs* 21, no. 3 (May-June 2002): 80-90.

Professionalism

1

Towards a New Concept of Professionalism: Being a Physician in Today's Healthcare System

Edward M. Spencer and Rebecca Bigoney

INTRODUCTION

Being a physician has, throughout time, had an aura of moral importance beyond the individual practitioner's personal moral code. This often nebulous but nevertheless real set of principles and virtues associated with being a physician has been maintained and enhanced through the medical education system and through the personal and professional relationships cultivated throughout physicians' practice careers. The primary tenet of this set of principles and virtues, whether stated or unstated, is generally understood by physicians and the larger society to be physicians' duty to advance whatever they feel is best for their individual patient(s). This understanding has been the basis for the trust necessary for an effective patient-physician relationship and is still believed by many to be the primary basis for this trusting relationship so necessary for optimum medical care.

Now, with changing ideas as to how healthcare should be defined, delivered, and paid for, physicians find that they are being asked (required?) to widen their moral perspective regarding what it means to be a physician, by considering issues once believed to be only business or management issues, and thus become bound by values that have to do with the "business" and "management" of the healthcare system. Many thoughtful physicians and others have worried that this expansion of the moral landscape that underlies what it means to be a physician may lead to contradictions, or at least a change in emphasis, away from traditional ideas concerning the importance of physicians' devotion to individual patients.[1]

Political and bureaucratic entities that have ties to the delivery and cost of healthcare (the Institute of Medicine), to practicing physicians (the American Medical Association), and to graduate medical education (the Accreditation Council for Graduate Medical Education), have made major recommendations, which, if fully implemented, will change the moral platform upon which physicians have traditionally stood, and thereby ultimately change what it means to be a physician.

The Institute of Medicine (IOM), during the past six years, has sponsored a series of three papers: the first, in 1999, documented the prevalence of medical mistakes;[2] the second, in 2002, defined quality in healthcare;[3] and the last, in 2004, recommended how to develop a comprehensive nationwide healthcare system.[4] The changes recommended include a strong endorsement of "evidence-based medicine," which supports the use of "best practices" that are derived from the medical literature to develop treatment protocols. The practice of evidence-based medicine should minimize variations in patient care, and, as a result, might reduce healthcare costs. However, some physicians speculate that its implementation may develop into "cookbook" medicine, which may have the undesirable effect of limiting the ability of physicians to individualize clinical recommendations, thereby undercutting the decision-making authority of doctors and their patients.[5] In addition, the American Medical Association (AMA) has been willing to change the *Code of Medical Ethics,* the repository of what it means to be an ethical physician, to accommodate the perceived wishes of society, even if the changes were made without full consideration of the possible effect on the traditional view of what it means to be a physician.[6] And finally, the Accreditation Council for Graduate Medical Education (ACGME) has instituted a number of requirements for resident training that greatly expands the areas that physicians must consider in their future practices and that change the concept of what it means to be a physician.[7]

In this chapter, we begin with a discussion of the traditional ideas of professionalism. Following this we will discuss the recent recommendations of the ACGME concerning the required competencies of residents in relation to knowledge of the healthcare system, of how to control healthcare costs, and of how to cooperate with other aspects of the system, including the business and management aspects of healthcare organizations. We will conclude by discussing some responses by physicians and the "system" that can possibly assure that a somewhat different, but nevertheless legitimate, moral landscape for the practicing physician can be developed and maintained, so that all can continue to understand what it means to be a physician in a moral sense.

TRADITIONAL PROFESSIONAL ETHICS

The more traditional clinician-based perspective concerning what it means to be a physician has been commonly called "professional medical ethics." In the past, this conceptualization of medical ethics has guided physicians when they encountered a situation described as an "ethical problem." Rather than focusing on rights or principles or on the system and its effects, this stream of medical ethics focuses largely on maintaining the professional integrity of the individual clinicians and their profession as they act in what they believe to be the best interest of each of their individual patients.

Traditional professional ethics has been externally documented in the form of professional codes. Within this tradition, codes, such as the American Medical Association's *Code of Medical Ethics,* are seen as the guiding beacons for the behavior of practitioners.[8] The codes supply advice and direction, both specific and general, concerning the proper manner of responding to a defined problem or circumstance. In addition, these codes define certain fundamental character traits that professional practitioners should exhibit, and insist that physicians maintain their devotion to the needs of their individual patients. Recently, the AMA *Code of Medical Ethics* has been expanded to include obligations to the larger society, thus paralleling the changes recommended by the IOM and the ACGME.[9]

INCLUSION OF PRINCIPLES PERTAINING TO BUSINESS PRACTICES AS A CONDITION FOR PROFESSIONALISM

The ACGME in 1999 endorsed a number of "competencies" that are expected to be met by all physicians completing an approved residency program. These competencies are related to all aspects of medical practice, including professionalism and systems-based practice. "Ethical practice," defined under "professionalism" by the ACGME, now includes "business practices" as a required area of knowledge.

The competency on professionalism states:

Residents must demonstrate a commitment to carrying out professional responsibilities, adherence to ethical principles, and sensitivity to a diverse patient population. Residents are expected to:

- demonstrate respect, compassion, and integrity; a responsiveness to the needs of patients and society that supersedes self-interest; accountability to patients, society, and the profession; and a commitment to excellence and ongoing professional development
- demonstrate a commitment to ethical principles pertaining to provision or withholding of clinical care, confidentiality of patient information, informed consent, and business practices
- demonstrate sensitivity and responsiveness to patients' culture, age, gender, and disabilities.[10]

The competency on professionalism details the virtues that physicians should exhibit when interacting with patients. There is no inconsistency between the professionalism competency and the traditional perception of medical ethics, since the competency describes the ideal behavior of physicians as being an obligation that is ultimately related to patient care. But the competency raises a whole new set of issues when business practices are included. To be sure, it may be that this inclusion was designed to address issues of fraud that the federal government has been so aggressively pursuing, as well as concerns raised by recent high-profile examples of unethical business practices in the corporate world, by requiring physicians to be honest and maintain a high degree of personal integrity when it comes to the "business" of care. But when we discuss business practices, we are addressing not only issues of billing, but the whole framework of relationships, systems, processes, and procedures that govern the way in which care is delivered and how it is compensated.

THE PHYSICIAN AND THE HEALTHCARE ORGANIZATION

Residents and physicians who are employees of healthcare organizations, or who act as independent professional staff members within the healthcare organization, or who are owners of their own practices, have their own sets of professional ethical obligations that are independent of whatever organization with which they are affiliated. These independent professional standards are maintained by professional associations and are codified into codes that are similar to the ones we have mentioned. To date, traditional professional standards have not been subject to control by organizational relationships or systems or procedures; nevertheless, they are important (maybe the most important) factors in the care provided to patients, and have a major effect on the business aspects of the organization. The tension between professional ethical mandates, particularly those that demand that the individual patient always comes first, and contractual obligations of the practice or healthcare organization, which often require attention to the needs of a group of "subscribers" rather than one individual patient, is an increasing source of conflict.

Can we flesh out principles that are associated with business practices so that they can be clear to individual physicians in the same manner as other industries? Can we assign rights and responsibilities in the same manner, so that the role of each actor in delivery of care is clear? In the healthcare context this may be difficult.

As businesses, healthcare organizations are distinctive from other industries in that the payer for services — be it an employer, governmental agency, or insurance company — is commonly not the "consumer" of the service provided. This means the major decisions about access to, and cost of, healthcare interventions are at least partially made by an entity that may be more interested in cost distributions than in the availability and quality of interventions for individual patients. In some instances patients, as recipients of care, have little clout to affect the availability of particular healthcare professionals from whom they can seek care. Nor can they be assured that they will have access to particular treatments and interventions, even though these interventions and treatments may be of proven value. In addition, patients are often vulnerable because of their illness. This vulnerability and the lack of the requisite knowledge to make truly informed decisions about the quality of care further assures that patients' decision-making authority is dependent on the particular organization and its values.

There is also a supply/demand asymmetry, since neither healthcare organizations nor their staff can ordinarily respond to all consumers' (patients') demands, in particular the demands of the uninsured, without threatening the economic survival of the organization. Moreover, some patients or groups of patients cannot pay for the healthcare they need or consume, while others pay for more than they consume.

These characteristics that distinguish healthcare organizations from other organizations make it difficult to point to the use of "business ethics" as a guide for professional obligations, although some attempts in this direction have been made.

Recent work in business ethics has depended heavily on a "stakeholder" concept as the basis for ethical organizational decision making. Under this model, it is the role of managers to weigh the varying obligations of the organization to the interested and affected stakeholders, which are usually believed to include stockholders, customers, payers (if different from customers), employees, contractual partners, the local community, and the larger society. After analyzing these obligations, a decision is made, based on the accepted values of the organization and the prioritized needs of its stakeholders.

Stakeholder theory sees itself as a normative theory that specifies reciprocal accountability relationships between stakeholders and the organization in question, that imports morally relevant standards for evaluating prioritization and decision criteria.[11] But there are problems, however, with using a traditional stakeholder concept to address organizational issues in physicians' practices or other healthcare organizations, which have to do with the aforementioned features of any organization that provides care. In addition, in many other businesses, the role of each stakeholder can be clearly identified. Along with this identification come mechanisms for each stakeholder (individual or group) to have appropriate decision-making authority in the aspects of the business that have an effect on the stakeholder as an individual and as a part of the organization. Under stakeholder theory, this authority is maintained by assigning rights and responsibilities based on the particular role of the individual. This is difficult in healthcare, because of the asymmetry in knowledge and power between the physician and patient, as well as the confusion of roles of the consumer (patient), the buyer or payer (employer, government, insurance provider, or managed-care organization), the healthcare professional, the manager (who is sometimes a healthcare professional as well), and the practice or healthcare organization itself, which often functions as provider, rationer, and controller of the delivery of healthcare services.[12] So how can residents and physicians reconcile the conflicting obligations and tensions detailed above?

RECONCILING CONFLICTING OBLIGATIONS

Some persons who have been interested in how these conflicts may be resolved have looked to healthcare organizational ethics. Organizational ethics recognizes that the healthcare organization is different from other industries, both in product and service, and in the way its services are delivered and reimbursed. It recognizes that business practices have normative characteristics and can influence the way in which care is delivered. But it also recognizes that neither business ethics nor traditional professional ethics (or clinical ethics), although they are important to maintaining healthcare organizations' excellence, is by itself able to address, let alone resolve, the complex and competing obligations of healthcare organizations and healthcare professionals.[13]

Organizational ethics focuses on the ethical climate of the organization, rationalizing that if the values of the healthcare organization are fully known and shared by its stakeholders, conflict is less likely. Moreover, it offers a mechanism by which unavoidable conflict can be resolved by appealing to the known values of the organization. Since most healthcare organizations have the goal of providing quality (or at least adequate) care, and since the goal of quality care cannot be divorced from the values that are associated with professionalism, this ensures that the traditional perspective of professionalism is both recognized and respected in any decision making. Organizational ethics, however, cannot guarantee that professionals' commitment to providing needed care for each individual, no matter the cost, will always be the primary determinant in each patient care decision. And the ACGME competency that is associated with systems-based practice may call into question whether organizational ethics, as it is currently understood, goes far enough in addressing the complexities that are associated with the delivery of quality healthcare services.

SYSTEM-BASED PRACTICE

The competency on systems-based practice requires that residents be aware of, and commit to, the goal of the larger system to provide quality, cost-effective care.

Residents must demonstrate an awareness of and responsiveness to the larger context and system of health care and the ability to effectively call on system resources to provide care that is of optimal value. Residents are expected to:

- understand how their patient care and other professional practices affect other health care professionals, the health care organization, and the larger society and how these elements of the system affect their own practice
- know how types of medical practice and delivery systems differ from one another, including methods controlling health care costs and allocating resources
- practice cost-effective health care and resource allocation that does not compromise quality of care
- advocate for quality patient care and assist patients in dealing with system complexities
- know how to partner with health care managers and health care providers to assess, coordinate, and improve health care and know how these activities can affect system performance.[14]

The previously mentioned competency on professionalism celebrates the traditional idea of the importance of physicians' character, but adds another: that residents must commit to the ethical principles of business practices. This competency adds another dimension to what it means to be a physician. Inevitable conflicts in the guiding ideals for the profession are the result, and some manner to address them is indicated.

The competency on systems-based practice expands the concept of "business practices," and, to some extent, attempts to maintain some of the traditional ideals by mentioning that physicians should advocate for quality patient care and assist patients in dealing with system complexities. If we see "business practices" as organizational systems or relationships or procedures or processes, then this competency can be viewed as an explanation or a description of what these business practices are, within which physicians will interact, and what outcomes they are required to produce. In the same way that the professionalism competency described the obligations of physicians, the systems-based practice competency describes the goal of the system, regardless of what form it takes, to provide care that is of optimal value. While recognizing the basic value of traditional professional ethics — to advocate for individual patients — it clearly also recognizes that physicians can only be patients' advocates within the context of a "system." This means that there can and likely will be numerous conflicts between the system and the professional mandate to advocate for quality care that revolves around the definition of "quality care."

The IOM, in its report *Crossing the Quality Chasm*, took a novel approach to viewing systems.[15] It took the view that the healthcare delivery system is a "complex adaptive system," or one that is made up of human beings who interact with each other within and through organizations.[16] A complex adaptive system is able to change, through its interactions, the goals of the system as well as the system itself. Obviously, such possibility for change depends upon significant integration throughout the system and a commitment from all aspects of the system to its values and goals.

Using this approach, the IOM suggested that if a healthcare delivery system, as a whole, subscribes to one goal: "All healthcare organizations, professional groups, and private and public purchasers should adopt as their explicit purpose to continually reduce the burden of illness, injury, and disability, and to improve the health and functioning of the people of the United States,"[17] and is guided by a few simple rules, the system would achieve this desirable goal.

Whether the IOM is right or not is an open question. But, if a system as a whole adopts the same goal, then there is a good chance that the system will achieve it. However, problems remain. In this case, the healthcare delivery system and all of its components must adopt this goal, and, if the delivery system adopts more than one goal, it must prioritize them similarly. If even one component of the system doesn't prioritize similarly, then, because it is a part of a complex adaptive system, the system will evolve in ways that can't be anticipated. This means that dissimilarities in priorities could produce outcomes that are inappropriate or that are directly counter to the IOM's desired goal. It is unlikely that the system as a whole will subscribe to the same set of goals and prioritize them similarly in the near term. Is it possible to apply the IOM's insights to a more micro system?

Since systems can be large or small, the IOM's insights are relevant when we think about the systems-based practice competency on a more micro level. There is no doubt that physicians or residents will be working within a complex adaptive system. Physicians, patients, as well as numerous other professionals and managers, are human beings who are coordinated together in a system that has business practices that are ideally designed to provide care at optimal value. But we know from the IOM's report that if one of the system's components does not share this goal, unanticipated consequences might emerge. From this perspective, the competency on systems-based practice could be seen as enlarging physicians' responsibilities. No longer are physicians required simply to base their interactions with patients on traditional professional ethics, but physicians are also required to ensure that system components all share the same goal or set of goals (prioritized similarly) and are coordinated together into business practices that further this goal or set of goals. Moreover, because it is a complex adaptive system, even if the system components share the same goal, the system's interactions can change the system itself, as well as its goal; thus, there is an additional responsibility to continuously evaluate the system and its interactions. Is this expectation reasonable? Is it reasonable to ask physicians, especially residents (who are preoccupied with learning), to accept responsibility for the outcomes of the system and, in addition, to make them responsible for continuously evaluating it? Are physicians, especially residents, so empowered that this is even a realistic expectation? Can this be either effective or efficient?

The ACGME competency on professionalism describes how physicians should interact with patients. It requires physicians to demonstrate respect, compassion, and integrity: responsiveness to patients' needs. Physicians may, in fact, exhibit all of these characteristics, but the business practices that define the system within which physicians practice may be characterized by disrespect, a lack of compassion and integrity, or a lack of responsiveness. In that case, surely the system will defeat the good intentions of physicians to provide optimal care. Or, consider whether or not the good intentions of a physician can be undermined, when one of the system's components does not share the physician's goals or interacts negatively with either patients or other system components.

In summary, there are three interrelated core elements of any system. First, there is the goal of the system; second, there are the business practices that define it; and third, there are the system components, all of which should adhere to the known values of the system. Each will have to be addressed for the system to function successfully, and the role of physicians in maintaining the successful functioning of the system is yet to be defined. It is obvious, however, that the traditional professional value relating to a pre-eminent obligation to an individual patient will not be possible under a systems-type practice. Instead, physicians must commit to different or expanded goals.

HEALTHCARE ORGANIZATIONAL ETHICS REVISITED

Healthcare organizational ethics addresses the goals of the system through its focus on the mission and values of the organization. Through this process, organizational ethics also impacts system design. Organizational ethics also seeks to influence system components and their interactions through its effect on the system components. If all components of the system share the organization's goals and values, then, assuming that its business practices reflect this, interactions among the systems components should also be consistent with the organization's goals and values. So organizational ethics addresses the three core elements of a system, but it can only address them internally.

Physicians and healthcare organizations work in the context of a larger system. The competency above recognizes this by requiring physicians to understand how their practice is affected by, and affects, the larger system. Organizational ethics, on the other hand, focuses on the internal goals and values of the organization. It acknowledges that organizations are different, and that they may have different values and goals. Although organizational ethics can exert some leverage on the system as a whole through its interactions with the external environment, it makes no claim to prescribing the values and goals of the macro system.

SYSTEMS-BASED PROFESSIONALISM

We began our discussion with a review of the traditional concept of what it means to be a physician: having certain desirable character traits and acting according to the perceived needs of individual patients. We have discussed how the competency on professionalism — by including an obligation for physicians to commit to the principles pertaining to business practices — adds another dimension to that concept. The competency on systems-based practice retains the ideal of physicians' role as a patient advocate, but explicitly recognizes that physicians are constrained by the system, and so their role may be limited or circumvented through the system.

We know that systems, whether we focus on the micro or macro level, have a goal; they have relationships — or, in this context, business practices — that define the system; and we know that interactions occur among system components within the context of these relationships. All three have the potential to prevent physicians from acting in their traditional role. Organizational ethics, as it is currently understood, may support the physicians' role in the micro context. But given the way systems function, it probably cannot affect the macro system to any significant degree.

But the systems-based practice competency has supplied a goal for both the micro and the macro systems — a goal that is not inconsistent with the goal supplied by the IOM. Providing care that is of optimal value can reduce the burden of suffering. As we struggle to implement (or possibly disrupt) the explicit and implicit goals of the IOM and the ACGME — in other words, to implement a system that will provide optimum care for all patients or, more realistically, for as many patients as possible — the question of the "best" role for physicians remains. And after that role has been defined, how should it be implemented? Should we scrap the traditional medical ethic that requires that the needs of the individual patient always take precedence over all else?[18] Should we develop a new and different professional ethics for physicians? Or should we in some manner try to integrate the traditional with the modern systems-based practice?

CONCLUSION

Obviously the ACGME would opt for integration, as would the IOM, the AMA, and most medical organizations. We know of no surveys of physicians that directly address this issue, and so cannot know the position of the physician community, but we guess that the majority of physicians would opt for an integrated approach. We also believe that the public at large is not yet ready to give up the ideal of the caring physician who is dedicated to the well-being of the patient.

But little attention has been given to this important issue. The ACGME has promulgated these competencies, but has yet to address how they (with other changes) will affect what it means to be a physician and how to develop a new expanded ethics for physicians.

We do not pretend to have the answers, but will offer a couple of suggestions. First, older physicians — particularly those teaching residents — need to understand the ramifications of these changes of the professional ethics of medicine and begin to discuss possible responses. The ACGME could and probably should be the sponsor of an educational endeavor for these teachers of future physicians. Secondly, until a new or expanded professional ethics is developed, the appropriate arena for resolution of ethical issues is the healthcare organization with which the physician is associated. This requires support and encouragement for the organization's organizational ethics program by physicians, and implies a willingness on the part of physicians to enter into discussions with other aspects of their organizations concerning matters that once may have been only in the purview of physicians. Local healthcare organizations will not always make the same decisions as physicians, but at least they offer a forum for discussion of professional ethical issues of importance to physicians and their patients.

What will it mean to be a physician in the future? We believe the profession must maintain a strong ethical base if it is to continue as more than a guild of talented technicians. To do this, each physician should continue to be an advocate for optimal care for his or her patients, while understanding that, due to scarce resources, patients may not always receive all of the interventions desired or needed. Physicians will need to understand the system, both micro and macro, and be able to use it for their patients' advantage, to the extent possible. And lastly, physicians must remember the long history of the profession, and use this knowledge of the profession's history to help determine its appropriate future direction. Even though the meaning is changing, it still should mean something important to be a physician.

ACKNOWLEDGMENT

The authors gratefully acknowledge Ann E. Mills for her contributions to the ideas developed in this chapter.

An earlier version of this chapter appeared in *Organizational Ethics: Healthcare, Business, and Policy*, volume 2, no.1 (Spring 2005). ©2005, University Publishing Group. Used with permission. All rights reserved.

NOTES

1. E.M. Spencer, "Professional Ethics," in *Fletcher's Introduction to Clinical Ethics,* ed. J.C. Fletcher, E.M. Spencer, and P.A. Lombardo (Hagerstown, Md.: University Publishing Group, 2005).

2. Committee on Quality of Health Care in America, Institute of Medicine, L. Kohn, J. Corrigan, and M. Donaldson, ed., *To Err is Human: Building a Safer Health System* (Washington, D.C.: National Academy Press, 2000)

3. Committee on Quality and Health Care in America, Institute of Medicine, *Crossing the Quality Chasm: A New Health System for the 21st Century* (Washington, D.C.: National Academy Press, 2001)

4. Committee on the Consequences of Uninsurance, Institute of Medicine, *Insuring America's Health* (Washington, D.C.: National Academy Press, 2004) *www.iom.edu/uninsured.*

5. O. Costantini et al., "Attitudes of Faculty, Housestaff, and Medical Students toward Clinical Practice Guidelines," *Academic Medicine* 74, no. 10 (1999): 1138-43.

6. The Council for Ethical and Judicial Affairs (CEJA), the group at the American Medical Association (AMA) that interprets the AMA's *Code of Medical Ethics* and issues "Current Opinions" on subjects of ethical importance, has attempted to consolidate bioethics and professional ethics by incorporating the viewpoint of contemporary bioethics into its code. AMA, CEJA, "Fundamental Elements of the Patient-Physician Relationship," in *Code of Medical Ethics* (Chicago, Ill.: AMA, 1996), xli-xliii.

In the early 1990s, CEJA added a new section to the *Code* called "Fundamental Elements of the Patient-Physician Relationship," and defined these fundamental elements in terms of the patients' rights rather than the more traditional physicians' obligations. AMA, CEJA, "Fundamental Elements of the Patient-Physician Relationship," in *Code of Medical Ethics* (Chicago, Ill.: AMA, 2002), 281-2.

In the 2002-2003 *Code of Medical Ethics,* "Fundamental Elements," as a part of the AMA *Code,* has been dropped, but continues as part of the "Current Opinions." In a number of its opinions on ethical issues, CEJA has addressed bioethics issues, has used the language of bioethics, and has appealed directly to contemporary bioethics for the foundational authority for the particular opinion. In doing so, it has gone beyond its mandated role of interpreting the *Code of Medical Ethics* and defining an ethical physician via opinions about the physician's obligations in specific circumstances.

In 1997, the AMA began an Ethics Standards Group to study and promote professionalism, which, on its surface, seems to be a response to a perceived need for some return to a traditional viewpoint. However, at the same time, the AMA initiated its "Institute for Ethics," which is an academic research and training center on ethics in healthcare that has had a bioethics viewpoint in its studies and educational activities. AMA, "Ethics Standards Group," in *Mission and Organization* (Chicago, Ill.: AMA, 2003), available at *www.ama.org*.

7. See *http://www.acgme.org/outcome//comp/compFull.asp*.

8. The present *Code of Medical Ethics* consists of three related parts: (1) "Principles of Medical Ethics," which is the fun-

damental statement of the core principles of the code; (2) "Current Opinions," which reflect the application of the principles to numerous specific ethical issues in medicine, and (3) "Reports," on issues of importance and interest prior to or concurrent with the issuance of an opinion.

The AMA's "Principles of Medical Ethics" are as follows:

PREAMBLE:

The medical profession has long subscribed to a body of ethical statements developed primarily for the benefit of the patient. As a member of this profession, a physician must recognize responsibility not only to patients, but also to society, to other health professionals, and to self. The following Principles adopted by the American Medical Association are not laws, but standards of conduct which define the essentials of honorable behavior for the physician.

I. A physician shall be dedicated to providing competent medical care, with compassion and respect for human dignity and rights.

II. A physician shall uphold the standards of professionalism, be honest in all professional interactions, and strive to report physicians deficient in character or competence, or engaging in fraud or deception, to appropriate entities.

III. A physician shall respect the law and also recognize a responsibility to seek changes in those requirements which are contrary to the best interests of the patient.

IV. A physician shall respect the rights of patients, colleagues, and other health professionals, and shall safeguard patient confidences and privacy within the constraints of the law.

V. A physician shall continue to study, apply and advance scientific knowledge, maintain a commitment to medical education, make relevant information available to patients, colleagues, and the public, obtain consultation, and use the talents of other health professionals when indicated.

VI. A physician shall, in the provision of appropriate patient care, except in emergencies, be free to choose

whom to serve, with whom to associate, and the environment in which to provide medical care.
VII. A physician shall recognize a responsibility to participate in activities contributing to the improvement of the community and the betterment of public health.
VIII. A physician shall, while caring for a patient, regard responsibility to the patient as paramount
IX. A physician shall support access to medical care for all people.

AMA, CEJA, *Code of Medical Ethics* (Chicago, Ill.: AMA, 2002), x-xi, p. xiv.

9. AMA, CEJA, see note 6 above.
10. ACGME, see note 7 above.
11. R.E. Freeman, *Strategic Management: A Stakeholder Approach* (Boston: Pitman Publishing, 1984); see also W. Evan and R.E. Freeman, "A Stakeholder Theory of the Modern Corporation: Kantian Capitalism," in *Ethical Theory and Business,* 3rd ed., ed. T. Beauchamp and N. Bowie (Englewood Cliffs, N.J.: Prentice-Hall, 1993), 101-5.
12. E.M. Spencer et al., *Organization Ethics in Healthcare* (New York: Oxford University Press, 2000).
13. Ibid.
14. ACGME, see note 7 above.
15. IOM, see note 3 above.
16. P. Plsek, "Redesigning Health Care with Insights from the Science of Complex Adaptive Systems," in IOM, *Crossing the Quality Chasm,* see note 3 above, pp. 310-33.
17. IOM, see note 3 above, p. 5.
18. A position that was never fully possible, as it would require the physician's attention to a very few patients. The inability to fully implement this mandate has been understood by physicians and patients alike, and, as long as the physician made an effort to render the best care possible under the circumstances, few were concerned.

2

Towards Systems-Informed Professionalism

Donna T. Chen, Ann E. Mills, and Patricia H. Werhane

INTRODUCTION

The Accreditation Council for General Medical Education (ACGME) competency on systems-based practice requires that residents "demonstrate an awareness of and responsiveness to the larger context and system of healthcare and the ability to effectively call on systems resources to provide care that is of optimal value." This competency requirement has caused some consternation among resident educators.[1] This is not surprising. Traditionally, physicians have been trained to think in terms of patients, not systems. To develop the knowledge, skills, and sensitivities required by the ACGME competencies will mean helping physicians to develop a mental model of their practice of medicine, and the systems that surround it, that is capable of embracing a systems perspective.

The ACGME goes further, however, than simply requiring physicians to recognize that the delivery of quality, cost-effective care depends on systems activities as well as on physicians' activities. The systems-based practice competency also suggests that physicians should "partner with . . . managers and . . . providers to assess, coordinate, and improve health care." Since healthcare depends on systems for delivery, this requirement, in effect, suggests that physicians should try to improve the healthcare systems within which they work. Together, the ACGME competencies on systems-based practice and professionalism —

which include both traditional professional values and a commitment to the ethical principles that pertain to business practices — spell out a set of knowledge, skills, and sensitivities that physicians will need to acquire to meet this challenge.

We begin this chapter with a discussion of systems generally and of the healthcare delivery system in particular. Then we move to a discussion of mental models, and how they can help us or can prevent us from seeing or understanding what is actually happening. We identify a management tool from the business literature that becomes the basis of a systems-informed perspective, a tool that can be used to help physicians to develop a mental model that informs systems-based practice, and we show how it captures the elements associated with the ACGME competency on systems-based practice.

We will argue throughout this chapter that a systems-informed perspective is just that — a systems-informed perspective. It can help inform the individual of the elements of a system, and it can help illustrate the interactions of a system. But if this perspective is used without the knowledge of the goals of a system and the values that those goals represent, it is incapable of helping or pointing physicians toward appropriate decision making.

The reverse is true as well. A systems-informed perspective, combined with the knowledge of and commitment to the goals of the system and its underlying values, might enable the individual to make appropriate decisions about systems-based practice, or to recognize when improvements to the system might be indicated.

In this context, the goal of the systems associated with healthcare delivery, as supplied by the ACGME competency on systems-based practice, is care of *optimal value,* or cost-effective quality care, and the associated values are the values supplied by the competency on professionalism. Goals, values, and their prioritization will supply direction when there is a conflict or uncertainty or confusion about a decision. An understanding of, and commitment to, the values associated with a new conceptualization of medical professionalism, one that reflects both traditional professional values and ethical principles associated with business practices combined with a systems-informed perspective moves the mental model we are developing from "systems-informed perspective" to "systems-informed professionalism," thus meeting the requirements of the two ACGME competencies under discussion.

But simply meeting the requirements of the competencies does not guarantee the delivery of healthcare that is high quality and cost-effective. Residents and other physicians have no control over larger systems, and most have very little control over systems at the organization level. Since this is the case, a mental model that requires physicians to consider the effects of decision making on other stakeholders, both individuals and groups, that in addition requires physicians to consider effects of resource usage, might heighten the conflicts physicians already feel in their practice, and end up doing a disservice to patients. Thus, we conclude that the delivery of quality, cost-effective care will require a consensus on the goals and values associated with care — and their prioritization — from all the components of the larger healthcare delivery system, and systems-informed professionalism provides a mental model for that as well.

SYSTEMS

All systems designed by humans, for use by humans, that use humans to fulfill their goals, whether they are micro systems (like a clinic or physician's practice) or a macro systems (like the whole of the healthcare delivery system), have common elements. Systems are designed for a purpose;[2] they are process driven; they utilize resources (like technology and human beings); and they must be at least minimally effective, or else they will not survive. Thus, a framework that incorporates a systems perspective must address all four elements: purpose, processes, resources needed, and effectiveness.

An important characteristic of any system is the degree of flexibility or rigidity it possesses. This distinction is fundamental and describes how the system is designed and how it responds to external or internal stimuli. For instance, a mechanical system will possess a high degree of rigidity. In such a system, we can predict in great detail the interaction of each of the parts in response to a given stimulus, since, in a purely mechanical system, pre-specified responses are always correct, and a correct response is always expected. For instance, a light switch is a mechanical system. If all parts are working correctly, when it is turned on, a light goes on. When deviation occurs (the light does not go on), it is unexpected and generally provokes study (is a fuse blown?) and action to prevent recurrence (replacing the fuse).[3] But systems that utilize the interactions of human beings in the achievement of their goals will exhibit at least a minimal degree of flexibility. The *degree* of flexibility will be determined by system designers in reference to the goals of the system, but no matter how rigidly it is designed, a system that relies on the interactions of humans to achieve its goals will reflect some degree of flexibility or adaptivity. This is because the interactions of human beings cannot always be controlled or predicted.

An adaptive system is one in which some (or all) parts of the system have the ability to respond to given stimuli in different and possibly unpredictable ways.[4] Adaptive systems have at least two characteristics that distinguish them from mechanical systems. First, the system itself has the ability to change through the interactions of its components. For instance, teams may find, through their interactions, a new and possibly more efficient way of communicating. Second, the goals or purposes of the system may change over time as the system responds in unpredictable ways to various stimuli. For instance, as a result of a discharge of a patient into a threatening environment, the team may add an additional goal to discharge procedures, perhaps the goal of ensuring that patients are discharged to a safe environment.

Systems also reflect the values deemed important for success. For instance, the designer of a fast food operation will value efficiency, reproducibility, and conformity to certain standards. If these values are not reflected in the processes of delivering fast food, then the system as a whole will not be effective and will probably fail. In a similar manner, healthcare delivery systems, whether these systems are hospitals, clinics, or practices, are or should be designed to reflect the values associated with healthcare, because these are the values that justify the support of the institution of healthcare by society, and they are the values that most healthcare professionals and the organizations they are associated with endorse.

MENTAL MODELS

Mental model is a concept developed by cognitive scientists, and used by Peter Senge and other organizational and systems theorists to help explain the human component of organizational and systems change, or lack thereof.[5] A mental model is a deeply held or ingrained assumption or generalization[6] that can take the form of patterns or images that influence how we understand the world. Mental models can be automated by pushing them into the unconscious. Ralph Stacey notes that this occurs during the process of becoming an "expert."[7]

Mental models both shape and influence how we experience the world. Indeed, we cannot experience *except* through mental models. Mental models are socially learned and incomplete, they can be distorting, and they are subject to change. Mental models are formed on the basis of past knowledge or experience and are used to understand the present so that decisions can be made and actions can be taken. They represent the ways that we constitute our experiences, the ways in which the brain stores, manages, and retrieves data selectively. Mental models offer benefits in the sense that they can be recalled and used rapidly and repeatedly. Furthermore, if they are shared, the need to communicate is lessened before a decision is made or an action is taken.

Although mental models offer benefits, they also bring serious or significant dangers. When they are unconscious, they are not being questioned. The very assumptions or generalizations used to create mental models may themselves be questionable, that is, individuals may make decisions or take action based on incorrect or problematic assumptions and generalizations. Or the situation may have changed since the mental model was developed. In these cases, mental models may cause us to filter out and miss what may be important elements of a given situation. Further, they may limit the possibilities we can envision to improve what we do.

Physicians have traditionally viewed their responsibilities primarily in terms of interactions with patients. This mental model may cause physicians to assume that their encounters with patients are isolated. Physicians who see an encounter or an interaction as isolated from the systems that surround the encounter may be blind to what is really happening to their patients. Donald Berwick offers an example. He points out that, in a systems-based practice, drawing tight boundaries between and among the roles of healthcare professionals might lead to a failure to cooperate or a failure to understand systemic implications, which could lead to a systems failure. Systems failures are not only wasteful, but can harm patients. Berwick points out that, from the viewpoint of the person served, the performance of a system "depends far more crucially on how elements work together than on how each element, in its role, performs separately."[8] This recognition forms the basis for the ACGME competency on systems-based practice. It is precisely why a wider perspective or mental model has been called for by the competencies.

A SYSTEMS-INFORMED MENTAL MODEL AND THE ELEMENTS OF A SYSTEM

To begin developing a systems-informed mental model, we borrow a management initiative from the business literature called the Balanced Scorecard, developed by Robert Kaplan and David Norton in the early 1990s.[9]

Kaplan and Norton introduced the Balanced Scorecard because they saw business organizations or companies as too reliant on financial considerations for making decisions. They were concerned that companies were at risk of failing if a financial perspective was used as the sole or dominant basis for decision making. They reason that although the financial viability of the company has to be sustained, it is elements reflect other important areas of the company that produce its outcomes. Since these other areas contribute to the success or failure of the company to achieve its goals, they too must be considered in decision making. Kaplan and Norton identify four interconnecting areas that are important to a company's long-run success, and they ask company leaders to consider the perspectives of each area, in decision making. These perspectives relate to issues associated with:

- financial considerations,
- internal processes,
- learning and growth, and
- customer expectations and satisfaction.

Kaplan and Norton see these areas as encompassing the whole of the business organization or company as it operates in its environment. The financial goals and the external constraints (the environment) of the company can be captured in the financial perspective. The internal business processes refer to the ways in which the company tries to achieve its goals; how it goes about accomplishing its mission. The "learning and growth" area Kaplan and Norton saw as relating to internal stakeholders, the people who implement the internal processes and their needs for growth in relation to desired company goals. The "customer" perspective is concerned with the expectations of the consumer or recipient of the company's products or services. In the business organization, the customer is generally the party who pays for the company's products or services, so whether or not the customer's expectations are being addressed is an important consideration for long-term stability or growth.

Kaplan and Norton believe that "success" from each perspective is critical to the long-term success of the business organization or company. If resources are not appropriately deployed to ensure success from each perspective, or, if one area is ignored, the company would suffer, and its long-term viability might be threatened. Thus, Kaplan and Norton hypothesize that company leaders, rather than relying solely on the financial perspective (or allowing it to dominate decision making), should develop a framework that included all four areas, so that an appropriate balance can be achieved.

Kaplan and Norton understood that all four perspectives are interconnected, and that a change in any one would affect all of the others. If resources are deployed to improve internal business processes, this may, in the short run, impact financial measures, learning and growth among employees, and customer satisfaction. For example, a company might initiate a quality improvement program in order to enhance its production or service capabilities. This program will impact the company's short-term profit and loss statements because the initial investment in quality improvement can be enormously expensive. [10] Associated with any such change might be a demand for changes in the behaviors of affected internal stakeholders,[11] which might require a specific educational intervention. Since a quality improvement program is generally designed to meet or exceed customer expectations, the perspective of the customer might change — although there is no guarantee that any of these changes will be the ones anticipated when the program was introduced.

Another example could be a change in the customers' expectations of the company due to a competitor's actions or a change in technology. This change might have profound implications for a company's internal business processes, its internal stakeholders, and its financial situation. Thus, because these areas are interconnected and because each is fundamental to the long-run success of the organization, Kaplan and Norton believed that organizational decisions need to take into account each of these four areas.

Kaplan and Norton understood that business organizations or companies are different — that, depending on their purpose, companies will prioritize differently. For instance, manufacturing firms will have different needs than service industries. They pointed out that the measures associated with each area could be tailored to suit the realities of each company. For example, performance measures will be different for industries that need their processes to be highly rigid than for industries that need flexibility in their processes to achieve appropriate outcomes

In the section under "Systems" in this chapter, we identify the elements that are common to systems that are designed and used by human beings — whether they are large or small. These elements — purpose, processes, resources needed, and effectiveness — are similar to the four areas described by Kaplan and Norton in their work on business organizations or companies.

Systems have a purpose — they are created and designed to achieve a goal. This corresponds to the "customer" perspective, because organizations cannot achieve long-term viability without customers. In most organizations, customers are consumers of products or services as well as payers for these products or services. Customers are the justification for an organization's existence. They give the organization a purpose.

Systems have processes that enable them to fulfill their purposes. An organization employs processes and procedures to achieve its goals. These processes correspond to the "internal processes" component. This area has to do with the way in which systems are designed and whether or not they are efficient and effective in producing desired outcomes. This area also has to do with the resources needed to build processes and maintain them.

Human systems generally require resources associated with technology, and, of course, human beings. But because human beings have special needs and because the interactions of human beings may change the system itself or its goals, we prefer, in exactly the same way as Kaplan and Norton, to distinguish between resources, and allow human beings a separate category so that the special needs of human beings who interact in different systems can be identified. This category, which we also call "learning and growth," can be used to target the special needs of humans as they endeavor to fulfill specific systems or organizational goals. This category, as Kaplan and Norton point out, can be tailored to suit the reality of the organization.[12] For instance, this category might be tailored to refer to and measure the special education or training humans need to excel in their functions. Or it may be that this category can be used to capture how well the individuals working in a system interact together. Or it can be used to inform organizational leaders about the culture and climate of the organization.

Finally, the system must be at least minimally effective in what it does, or it will not survive. This is akin to the financial perspective. Any organization that is not financially viable cannot exist in the long run. Thus, this framework gives us a tool to use to examine the impact of decisions on all facets of the system or organization. It enables us to acquire a "systems-informed" perspective.

In figure 2.1 we demonstrate how the areas described in the Balanced Scorecard equate to the elements of a system.

FROM "SYSTEMS-INFORMED PERSPECTIVE" TO "SYSTEMS-INFORMED PROFESSIONALISM"

A systems-informed mental model challenges residents to think through the implications of an action or decision in these multiple dimensions. Its precise intent *is* to challenge existing mental models, which divorce the professional from the interactions of the system within which he or she functions. But simply having a systems-informed perspective does not guarantee that appropriate decisions will be made. Without goals, the values that reflect them, and their prioritization, a system will almost

LINKING SYSTEM ELEMENTS AND THE AREAS DESCRIBED IN THE BALANCED SCORECARD

Elements of a System	Purpose	Processes	Resources	Effectiveness
The Four Perspectives of the Balanced Scorecard	Customer	Internal Processes (including design and resources required, excepting human beings)	Learning and Growth (the special needs of humans)	Financial

Figure 2.1.

certainly be chaotic, and ultimately may cease to exist. This is especially true in human systems. Without agreed-upon goals, values, and their prioritization, persons might assign priorities in conflicting ways, or they may have entirely dissimilar values and goals.[13] This will almost certainly generate conflict and inconsistent results. In such a case, the system will, at best, be inconsistent in achieving its goals. Thus, effective systems, especially those whose effectiveness depends on the interactions of humans, require a consensus on goals, values, and their prioritization. In the context of healthcare, the ACGME requires that physicians commit to the values associated with a new conceptualization of professionalism, one which includes traditional professional values and ethical principles associated with business practices. If this commitment is made by a physician working within systems, then a systems-informed perspective will need to move towards a mental model that is characterized by systems-informed professionalism.

As Berwick observes, physicians' practice of medicine can also be considered through a systems-informed perspective.[14] Physicians' practice is dependent upon interacting systems that operate on a micro basis as well as on a macro basis. To be effective, physicians must understand the systems within which they work. But, even if physicians have committed to the values associated with a professionalism that reflects traditional professional values and the ethical principles that are associated with business practices, if the systems with which the physicians interact reflect different values, inconsistent results will be achieved. For instance, there are procedures and processes that are followed both before and after physicians see patients. If these procedures and processes do not reflect the values associated with professionalism, they will affect patients' perception of the quality of care they receive. Echoing Berwick, will it matter to patients if they have a good experience with their physician, if the patients are harmed through inattention in whatever follow-up care they may need?

ETHICAL CLIMATE AND SYSTEMS-INFORMED PROFESSIONALISM

We can think of systems as being large or small. Often, we think of systems in isolation, but, in reality, as in a healthcare organization or practice, various systems interact together to achieve an outcome. For instance, a given patient may be referred to other practices, may require various laboratory tests or interventions, or may require follow-up care. Each system interacts with another and each might help or prevent the other from achieving its purpose.

As noted earlier, systems can exhibit varying degrees of rigidity or flexibility. Ann Mills and Mary Rorty argue in their chapter, "Business Practices, Ethical Principles, and Professionalism," that, in the context of healthcare, systems that are designed to promote medical professionalism must be flexible enough to support a physician's professional judgment. But the very flexibility required to support professionalism might endanger appropriate outcomes. Therefore, it is necessary to find some "glue" or consistent factor throughout interacting systems so that one system does not impede the performance of another. In a healthcare organizational context, this "glue" can be a positive ethical climate.[15]

As described more fully in the introduction to this book and in Paul Clark's essay, "The Ethical Climate: Can Organization Ethics Programs Influence Management Initiatives?" a positive ethical climate has at least two important characteristics. First, a positive ethical climate embodies a set of shared values that reflect societal norms for what the organization should value; how it should prioritize its mission, vision, and goals; and how the organization and the individuals associated with it should behave. Second, it is an organizational culture in which the mission and vision of the organization inform expectations for professional and managerial performance, *and* in which the mission and vision are implemented in the actual practices of the organization, in part because the mission and vision reflect shared values.[16] One of the most important characteristics of an organization with a positive ethical climate is congruence of values: agreement on priorities among organizational leaders, congruence of values between leaders and internal constituents, and compatibility of organizational values with the larger social environment in which the organization operates. [17]

If the various functional units of a healthcare delivery system and the individuals associated with them agree that their activities and decisions will reflect the goal of quality, cost-effective care, then a consensus can be achieved as to how decisions and activities will take place. That consensus can be formed around the values associated with a medical professionalism that reflects traditional professional values, as well as the ethical principles associated with business practices, because, in a healthcare context, "quality" is not meaningful unless the values associated with medical professionalism are reflected. Thus, any healthcare organization that states that its mission is the delivery of care of high quality must make a commitment to these values.

We are talking here about the possibility of the ethical climate reducing, not eliminating, conflict. Conflict *will* occur. Men and woman of integrity and intelligence will perceive different solutions to the problems of providing cost-effective quality care, and this conflict will be seen (and is seen) in both the micro and macro delivery context.[18] But an agreement on goals and the values they reflect provides an appropriate ethical climate in which to negotiate solutions, and a perspective characterized by systems-informed professionalism cannot be completely effective without such a climate.

The ACGME is asking physicians to commit to the values associated with a new conceptualization of professionalism and to develop a systems-informed perspective — taken together, the ACGME is asking physicians to develop a perspective that is characterized by systems-informed professionalism. This involves solving problems that are associated with healthcare systems and improving healthcare systems in the context of the values that are associated with this new conceptualization of professionalism, which reflects both traditional medical professional values and the ethical principles associated with business practices. If these values are absent in the healthcare systems within which physicians work, and if there is no possibility of negotiating their inclusion, then asking physicians to commit to this perspective may be a meaningless undertaking. Certainly, a systems-informed perspective will enable physicians to understand the healthcare systems within which they are embedded. But if physicians are prevented by the systems from making decisions on the basis of a professionalism that reflects traditional professional values and ethical principles associated with business practices, then why ask or require physicians to commit to these values? Effectively, physicians would be powerless to make decisions based on them. In this situation, when physicians who work within systems are unable to make decisions based on a professionalism that reflects both traditional professional values and ethical principles associated with business practices, they may be tempted to revert to a mental model that sees encounters with patients as isolated events — a mental model in which physicians are able to maintain a sense of traditional "professionalism," but one that is ultimately incompatible with systems-based practice, and, without the support of the system, might ultimately be a compromised or false sense of professionalism. Maintaining a perspective that is characterized by systems-informed professionalism may allow physicians to recognize the sort of situation in which it might be best for them to leave the system.

SYSTEMS-INFORMED PROFESSIONALISM: A REPRESENTATION

Our conception of systems-informed professionalism requires physicians to expand their mental model beyond a series of one-on-one patient encounters. This shift in mental models is akin to the need for companies to broaden their view of success beyond the financial perspective. Physicians must recognize that they work in systems, and they must understand the important elements that are associated with systems and how these elements interact to produce the system's goals. Physicians must understand that the system will not survive without an appropriate balance between its various elements. But this is not enough. A framework can identify the important elements of systems and show their interactions — but a framework alone cannot guide decision making. For this we must have goals and values.

In our framework (see figure 2.2), we have modified the generic model supplied by Kaplan and Norton and have placed the patient and community first. This highlights the fact that it is the patient, and the community of potential patients, who are the consumers of healthcare, and the reason that a healthcare delivery system exists in the first place. The fact that the patient and community are not generally those who pay for healthcare products and services is one the distinguishing features of the healthcare system. Since consumers and payers are ordinarily not the same party, their expectations will be different. Nevertheless, one of the key features of professionalism in healthcare requires that healthcare professionals elevate patients' interests above their own interests. This requirement has not changed. So neither physicians nor healthcare organizations can claim to be profession-

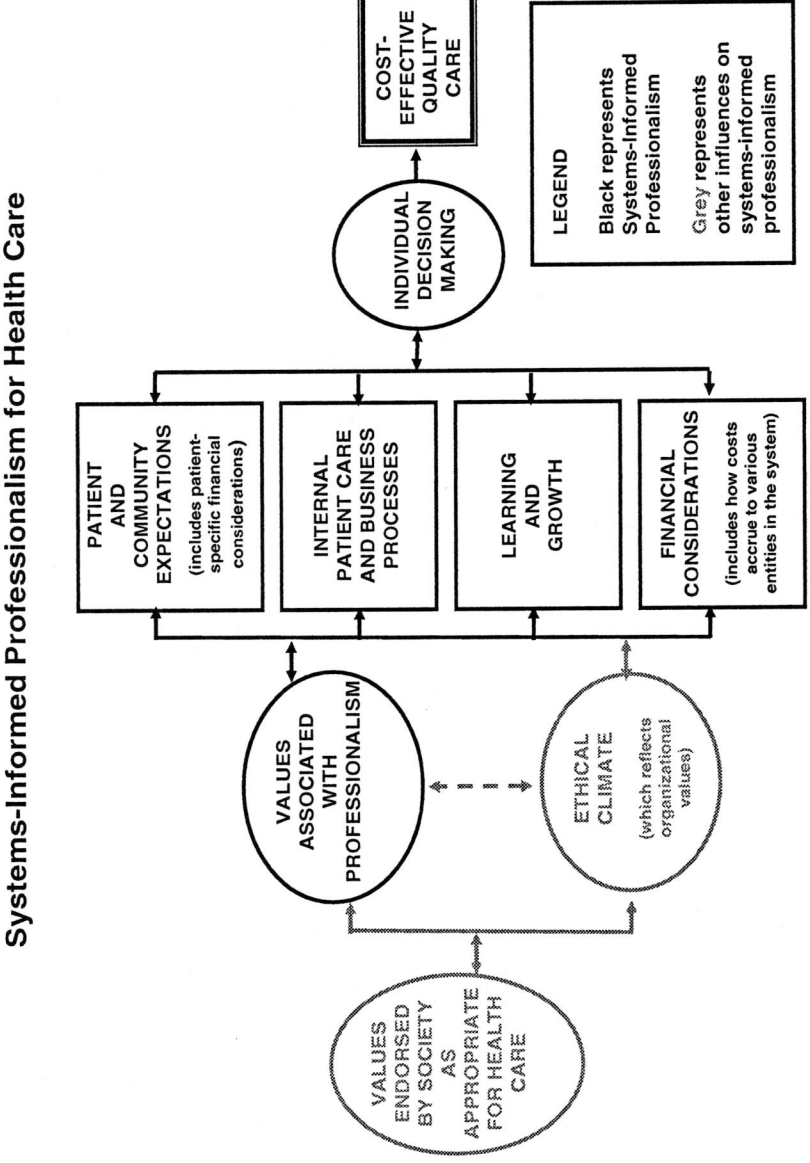

Figure 2.2.

als or professional organizations unless their first priority is the patient and the community. Nevertheless, being sensitive to the needs of patients may also require physicians to consider how patients may be affected by the healthcare systems, including insurance or medical plans. Even though patients are generally not the primary payers for healthcare goods and services, plans determine in large part the type and amount of care that patients receive. Thus, in contemplating how to achieve the best possible outcome for patients, physicians or healthcare organizations may need to consider patient-specific financial information.

We have chosen to designate "internal processes" as "internal patient care and business processes" to highlight that *both* are necessary processes in healthcare delivery systems, and excellent functioning is required of both. In our model, "learning and growth" refers to the specific knowledge, attitudes, and skills required of physicians by the ACGME competencies — not just learning them now, but continuing to sharpen them and developing a worldview that recognizes that, as the systems of care change, adjustments in the activities and obligations required to fulfill the commitments associated with professionalism may also change.

We have placed "financial considerations" at the bottom to illustrate that the financial viability of the healthcare organization is both the foundation for and the result of excellence in the other three areas. Success in developing the processes and skills for excellent patient care requires financial support, and it has financial consequences. So financial viability requires physicians to understand that costs accompany the provision of care, and that costs will accrue to one or more entity in the healthcare system. This represents a deviation from the generic model of Kaplan and Norton, in that, from one perspective, payers can be considered "consumers," which implies that their requirements and expectations should be the foremost consideration in decision making. While patient care *is* the justification for the healthcare system, and so should be the foremost consideration in decision making, this should not prevent physicians or healthcare organizations from considering requirements for cost-effectiveness. This is equally true for for-profit and not-for-profit healthcare organizations. Financial viability and cost-effectiveness are always goals of both kinds or organizations, even when profitability, per se, is not an issue. This is precisely the reason why a broader perspective, such as systems-informed professionalism, is needed — so that the requirements of patients and their payers can be reconciled in the delivery of quality, cost-effective care.

The values associated with professionalism, which now include attention to both traditional professional values and the ethical principles associated with business practices, are the filter through which these four areas — "patient and community expectations," "internal patient care and business processes," "learning and growth," and "financial considerations"— can be examined and evaluated so that individual decision making is aligned with these values. We recognize that, ultimately, reflecting these values in any one individual or system is not enough. They must be reflected in *all* of the systems with which physicians interact. But because no one individual or organization can control all of the elements of the larger delivery system, we must be satisfied, for the meantime, with looking for a consensus on values by persons associated with the healthcare organization, a mid level system.

To be sure, healthcare organizations do not control decisions made in the larger delivery system. But they can control their responses to these decisions and they can create, as Evan DeRenzo suggests in her essay, "Individuals, Systems, and Professional Behavior" a "morally safe environment" or a positive ethical climate for their residents and other physicians. Thus, in our framework, the ethical climate supports the values that are associated with professionalism. This allows these values to be reflected by decisions made by the individual within the context of a system that may result in achieving the goals of the competencies — quality, cost-effective care.

SYSTEMS-INFORMED PROFESSIONALISM AND THE ACGME COMPETENCIES

The competencies proposed by the ACGME Outcome Project call for a new mental model that is capable of allowing physicians to see the elements of a system, to understand the interactions of the elements, to appreciate the impact of the system on them as well as the impact of their actions on the system, and to recognize that they are a critical part of the system. We believe a systems-informed perspective, built on the Balanced Scorecard, accomplishes this. Can this framework reflect the elements as-

The ACGME Competency on Systems-Based Practice and the Elements of a System-Informed Perspective for Health Care

	Patient and Community Expectations (includes patient-specific financial considerations)	Internal Patient Care and Business Processes	Learning and Growth	Financial Considerations (includes how costs accrue to various entities in the system)
Residents must demonstrate an awareness of and responsiveness to the larger context and system of health care and the ability to effectively call on system resources to provide care that is of optimal value.	X	X	X	X
Residents are expected to				
• understand how their patient care and other professional practices affect other health care professionals, the health care organization, and the larger society and how these elements of the system affect their own practice	X	X		X
• know how types of medical practice and delivery systems differ from one another, including methods of controlling health care costs and allocating resources		X		X
• practice cost-effective health care and resource allocation that does not compromise quality of care	X	X		X
• advocate for quality patient care and assist patients in dealing with system complexities	X	X		
• know how to partner with health care managers and health care providers to assess, coordinate, and improve health care and know how these activities can affect system performance		X	X	

Figure 2.3.

sociated with the ACGME competency on systems-based practice? Below, in figure 2.3, we show how this is possible.

As discussed earlier, the four elements of any systems decision that should be considered are:

- the desired end result of the decision on the customer, who is the patient,
- the implications associated with internal business or patient care practices,
- the impact on the people who need to carry out the decision, and
- the financial implications of the decision.

The four areas of the systems-informed perspective,

- patient and community expectations,
- internal patient care and business processes,
- learning and growth, and
- financial considerations,

allow physicians to recognize the four elements that are considered to be important to the successful functioning of any system, whether it is a micro system, or large, complex, mid level system, like a healthcare organization.

By now it should be clear that this perspective can accommodate *all* of the ACGME competencies.[19] The competency on "practice-based learning and improvement" is process driven, in that it involves investigation and evaluation of patient care, appraisal and assimilation of scientific evidence, and improvements in patient care. Practice-based learning also requires critical self-evaluation. Thus, it also has implications for "learning and growth." The competency on "interpersonal and communication skills" may be considered a "learning and growth" skill, as can the competency on "medical care." The "patient care" competency directs attention to the expectations of the patient, the customer of care. All of the ACGME competencies reflect some aspect of patient care or business practices. If meaningful decisions are to be made, the goals and values associated with the competency on professionalism must drive decision making in each of the areas. Thus, it is possible to view each of the competencies as components of appropriate system performance, as shown below in figure 2.4.

A Comprehensive View of the ACGME Competencies and the Elements of a Systems-Informed Perspective for Health Care

The ACGME Competencies	Elements of a Systems-Informed Perspective for Health Care			
	Patient and Community Expectations (includes patient-specific financial considerations)	Internal Patient Care and Business Processes	Learning and Growth	Financial Considerations (includes how costs accrue to various entities in the system)
Patient Care	X	X		X
Medical Knowledge		X	X	
Practice-Based Learning and Improvement		X	X	
Interpersonal and Communication Skills		X	X	
Systems-Based Practice	X	X	X	X

Values Associated with Professionalism

Figure 2.4.

SUMMARY AND CONCLUSION

This chapter introduces the idea of systems-informed professionalism, with which we hope to challenge existing mental models of care that see professional medical responsibilities as beginning and ending with individual encounters and interactions with patients. We are not down-playing the importance of physician-patient interactions, which remain central to and define the role of physicians in the healthcare system. Rather, we are asking physicians to see these interactions in the context of a system, to understand that the successful delivery of care depends as much on systems as it does on physician-patient interactions.

We see the development of a mental model that is characterized by systems-informed professionalism as important to the delivery of quality, cost-effective care. But there are caveats. Adopting this model does not mean that all conflict can be avoided. Even within a systems-based practice, the patient must take primacy. Physicians must prioritize their activities in relationship to their patients. For instance, they must prioritize patient activities and required documentation, which may generate conflict in other systems. But, in the language of business, these are operational problems, which can generally be resolved, if the components of the systems, as well as interconnecting systems share the same goals and values and prioritize their goals and values similarly. It is when systems and their components do not share the same values and goals, or when they prioritize them differently, that one can predict that results will not be optimal, and that the individuals involved will be neither happy nor satisfied.

In the current healthcare environment, we cannot presuppose the alignment of values that characterizes a positive ethical climate in a healthcare organization, or that would characterize a well-integrated and excellently functioning healthcare system. Physicians do not control larger systems. They do not control the larger delivery system and they do not control, or even have much influence over, the healthcare organizations with which they are associated. The goals and values associated with these larger systems may not mirror the goals and values that professionalism requires of physicians. Hence, there may be little basis for conflict resolution when interacting systems are designed to produce dissimilar goals and reflect different values. But any significant improvement in the quality of healthcare in the US involves and often begins with the physicians who are its primary agents. This is reflected in the ACGME's desire to train physicians to provide excellent patient care within complex systems and to work to improve those systems, particularly to help ensure that the systems reflect values that are associated with medical professionalism.

ACKNOWLEDGMENTS

We gratefully acknowledge the advice and comments of Mary V. Rorty and Bradford B. Worrall in the preparation of this manuscript. Donna Chen is supported in part by NIMH grant 1P20MH071897.

NOTES

1. G. Ogrinc et al., "A Framework for Teaching Medical Students and Residents about Practice-based Learning and Improvement, Synthesized from a Literature Review," *Academic Medicine* 78, no. 7 (2003): 748-58.
2. A. Laszlo and S. Krippner, "Systems Theories: Their Origins, Foundations and Development," in *Systems Theories and a Priori Aspects of Perception,* ed. J. Scott (Amsterdam: Elsevier, 1988), 51.
3. P. Plsek, "Redesigning Health Care with Insights from the Science of Complex Adaptive Systems," in *Crossing The Quality Chasm: A New Health System for the 21st Century* (Washington D.C.: National Academy Press; 2001): 309-23.
4. Ibid., 311.
5. P. Senge, *The Fifth Discipline: The Art and Practice of the Learning Organization* (New York: Doubleday, 1990.)
6. P. Werhane, *Moral Imagination and Management Decision Making* (New York: Oxford University Press 1999), 11-2.
7. R.D. Stacey, *Strategic Management and Organisational Dynamics: The Challenge of Complexity* (New York: Prentice Hall, 2003.)
8. D. Berwick, "Crossing the Boundary: Changing Mental Models in the Service of Improvement," *International Journal for Quality in Health Care* 10, no. 5 (1998): 435-41.
9. R.S. Kaplan and D.P. Norton, *The Balanced Scorecard: Translating Strategy into Action* (Boston, Mass.: Harvard Busi-

ness School Press, 1996).

10. P.S. Pande, R.P. Neuman, and R.R. Cavanagh, *The Six Sigma Way: How GE, Motorola, and Other Top Companies Are Honing their Performance* (New York, N.Y.: McGraw Hill, 2000).

11. J. Detert, R.G. Schroeder, and J.J. Mauriel, "A Framework for Linking Culture and Improvement Initiatives in Organizations," *Academy of Management Review* 25, no. 4 (October 2000): 850-63.

12. Kaplan and Norton, see note 9 above.

13. A.E. Mills, M.V. Rorty, and P.H. Werhane, "Complexity and the Role of Ethics in Health Care," *Journal of Complexity Issues in Organizations and Management* 5, no. 3 (October 2003): 13-21.

14. See note 8 above, p. 438.

15. See note 13 above.

16. E.M. Spencer et al., *Organization Ethics for Healthcare Organizations* (Oxford: Oxford University Press, 2000).

17. J. Denis, L. Lamothe, and A. Langley, "The Dynamics of Collective Leadership and Strategic Change in Pluralistic Organizations," *Academy of Management Journal* 44 (2001): 809-37.

18. J.C. Robinson. "The End of Managed Care," *Journal of American Medical Association* 285, no. 20 (May 2001)): 2622-8.

19. The ACGME General Competencies are included in an appendix to this volume.

3

The Ethical Climate: Can Organizational Ethics Programs Influence Management Initiatives?

Paul A. Clark

INTRODUCTION

Organizational ethics programs seek to "produce a positive ethical climate, where organizational policies, activities, and self-evaluation mechanisms integrate patient, business, and professional perspectives in consistent and positive ventures that articulate, apply, and reinforce an organization's mission in value-creating activities throughout the organization."[1] *Ethical climate* is the shared set of understandings about correct behavior and how employees perceive ethical issues will be handled.[2] As part of organizational culture, the ethical climate helps translate an organization's mission into daily work, determines viable actions, and decides what behaviors will be rewarded or criticized.[3] In this way, the ethical climate influences employees' interrelationships, the quality of work life, employees' satisfaction, and management outcomes.[4]

Some, but not all, healthcare systems or organizations have formal organizational ethics programs and/or organizational ethicists. Nevertheless, since the ethical climate influences value-creating activities, especially in service industries where interactions between stakeholders are reflected in the processes employed by organizations to achieve their goals and the outcomes produced by these processes, in organizations without a formal organizational ethics program and/or an organizational ethicist, someone or ones should be responsible for and committed to attending to the positive ethical climate.

Traditionally, healthcare ethics has remained within exclusive domains — clinical- or patient-centered ethics, professional ethics, or business ethics. Organizational ethics programs establish a process to integrate these perspectives, and the perspectives of all legitimate stakeholders, with the goal of improving the overall ethical climate.

Stakeholders' interests will sometimes overlap, and sometimes they will be mutually exclusive.[5] An organization's outcomes may reflect a failure to distribute scarce resources justly if the perspective of one stakeholder dominates decision making. Thus senior managers, in any organization, have an extraordinary duty to ensure proper and appropriate allocation of resources among stakeholders whose interests may be mutually exclusive. The challenge is to make these distributive decisions appropriately, which may involve appeal to some other goal, or metric, or value, rather than relying solely on the financial perspective.[6]

A similar challenge gave birth to the Balanced Scorecard (BSC) management initiative in the early 1990s. At the threshold of the knowledge-based economy, Robert S. Kaplan and David P. Norton saw organizations as so overly reliant on financial measures that their competitive and decision-making abilities were impeded.[7] Financial measures did not capture an organization's intangibles: employees' skills, competencies and morale; intellectual capital and information technology; internal operating systems and processes; innovation; customer relationships and loyalty; and the political, regulatory, and community environment. Failures or changes in any of the aforementioned areas could derail an organization's strategy and significantly harm its financial outcomes. Any large, complex organization attempting to achieve a broad range of goals requires the strategic integration of an equally broad set of performance measures to indicate whether or not it was achieving them. This problem was solved through the BSC approach.

At a recent conference on organizational ethics in healthcare, Patricia Werhane suggested that a BSC framework can operate to achieve an appropriate, and maybe just, equilibrium between competing interests.[8] Can a process that is concerned with the goal of a positive ethical climate help in the design and execution of a management initiative, specifically the BSC?

THE BALANCED SCORECARD

The BSC is a management approach that offers executives the ability to combine strategic objectives with operations and performance data for organizational evaluation and improvement.[9] Since Kaplan and Norton developed the original BSC approach in 1992, numerous very large and diverse organizations, such as 3M, Chase, Mobil, and AT&T, have used the framework associated with it to achieve radical performance improvement.[10]

The original BSC framework delineated four interdependent strategic perspectives or quadrants: financial, internal business processes, learning and growth, and customer. Associated with these quadrants are specific measures that inform management how well (or not) an organization achieves its goals. According to Kaplan and Norton, typical measures associated with these quadrants will include:

- Financial perspective — revenue growth, cost reduction, market share, stock price, et cetera.
- Internal business processes — quality measures, process measures, et cetera.
- Learning and growth — employees' satisfaction, skills learned, et cetera.
- Customers' perspective — customers' satisfaction, loyalty, and so forth.

Measures that may be associated with healthcare organizations will be similar, but will include those specific to the industry and individual healthcare organization. For instance, associated with the BSC financial perspective, a healthcare organization may include measures such as labor cost as a percentage of revenue, or total cost per adjusted discharge. Measures associated with internal business practices may include items such as admit-to-bed placement or the ratio of registered nurses to bed. Employee growth measures may include staff education or employees' satisfaction, and the customers' satisfaction perspective may include measures of patients' satisfaction. But in every organization, successful implementation of the BSC management framework depends on several critical factors. Assuming that the organization's mission, vision, values, and/or strategy are successfully identified and articulated, the first step in the BSC approach is deciding what to measure; the wrong measures or too many measures may lead to demoralization or failure to achieve the organization's goals. In addition, the measures must be scientifically reliable and valid, as well as accurately reflective of the overarching vision, mission, values, and/or strategy. They also must be relevant enough to be associated with other critical but relatively less visible variables (for example, improvements in employees' satisfaction correlate with lower turnover, fewer missed days, and greater productivity; improvements in loyalty tend to eventually spur increases in volume; et cetera).

The success of the scorecard will depend heavily on the effectiveness of communicating what is being measured and the results of measurement. It will also depend on how frequently (daily, weekly, biweekly, or monthly) measurement mechanisms are used.[11]

OPPORTUNITY FOR INFLUENCE FOR ORGANIZATIONAL ETHICS PROGRAMS

MISSION, VISION, AND VALUES

One set of measures cannot fit all organizations, as missions, values, and even definitions of success diverge among industries and the organizations associated with them.[12] Therefore, for organizational ethicists and others committed to creating a positive ethical climate, the first opportunity for influence is to identify and articulate the organization's mission and values. These will be the foundation on which the scorecard rests,[13] and so will ultimately drive decision making in the organization.[14] In the BSC, measurement is linked to mission and values. Thus, the BSC ensures that the organization's mission and values are integrated into senior managements' thinking and decision making.

Perhaps the most important goal of the BSC is to capture the perspectives of all the organization's major stakeholders. Organizational functions that are not represented in the BSC will tend to decline in value, leadership support, and management priority, and of course, resources. Therefore, another opportunity for influence for organizational ethicists is to ensure that all important functions are represented in the BSC.

The Ethical Climate

Although most ethical dilemmas arise when values conflict,[15] most healthcare executives don't consider conflicting values or interests to be issues involving "ethics."[16] It is common among administrators and managers, and not just in healthcare, to view most decisions as "value-neutral" or "business decisions." But after nominal analysis, one sees that every decision is laden with values that may negate the moral agency of the individual or organization.[17] The contents of an organization's BSC represent what the organization values, and, because it is articulated, these values should be clear to all stakeholders.

MEASUREMENT

Organizational ethicists and others interested in ensuring a positive ethical climate might also influence *what* is measured and *how* it is measured. They may be able to help decision makers align the BSC measures with the values imbued in the mission, vision, values statements, as well as the organization's strategies. A focus on specific measures defines the meaning of values like "quality," "excellence," "customer satisfaction," and other relatively elusive ideals. For example, quality can be assessed by patients' satisfaction with their involvement in treatment decisions.[18] Including this measure in the BSC and assigning a benchmark to it may later result in performance improvement efforts, for instance, communication skills training, or decision-making aides, or patient education materials.

In implementing a BSC performance measurement system, the Mayo Clinic (Rochester, Minnesota) learned that people will perform and manage to exactly what it is that is being measured.[19] What gets measured and how it is measured will define where healthcare managers concentrate efforts for improvement, including allocating scarce resources to ensure and promote it.

Any hope of improving performance that one seeks to achieve through the BSC depends upon sound measurement methodology. Appropriate and accurate measurement is important to not only prevent organizational misdirection (achievement of outcomes not aligned with the organization's values), but to prevent miscarriages associated with managerial accountability. Since the entire purpose of the BSC approach rests upon driving healthcare management decisions — and accountability for them — based upon the values of the organization and measurable results, measurement methodology matters. Gaming measurement or selecting measures with methodologies that ultimately render them meaningless can be tempting. As guides in mission, vision, and values, organizational ethicists may find themselves arbiters in BSC measurement decisions. But being involved in these decisions will necessitate an understanding of performance measurement methodologies. For example, one must consider the source of the data, its relevance, whether or not it is feasible to obtain, whether or not it is objective or subjective, and whether or not it will give us a measure that can be validly used.[20] For example, poor patient satisfaction methodology can result in misleading or entirely inaccurate results. Consequently, hospitals could:

- Waste scarce resources on futile improvement initiatives;
- Mistakenly censure healthcare professionals;
- Issue undeserved rewards;
- Fail to recognize significant service delivery problems;
- Set inappropriate goals;
- Fail to meet Joint Commission on Accreditation of Healthcare Organizations (JCAHO) accreditation requirements.

There are other good reasons to measure performance and to insure its appropriateness. In the private insurance world, 31 separate sponsors of pay-for-performance initiatives already affect over 20 million enrollees.[21] As Charles Denham notes, "The current no-margin, no-mission era in health care is coming to an end. It is giving way to a new no-outcome, no-income era. Revenue will no longer be automatic; it will be increasingly linked to verifiable performance."[22]

DISSEMINATION OF THE VALUES ASSOCIATED WITH THE BSC

As one of the few agents in a healthcare delivery organization that can easily cross professional and departmental borders, organizational ethicists are in a unique position to encourage the dissemination of the values associated with the BSC to all corners of the organization. Since the BSC is intended to have an overall effect on the organization, and since it delineates the organization's mission, vision, and values, every person in the organization should be aware of and evaluate their activities based upon it. Internal service departments, such as supply management, finance, and, especially, human resources, are not immune from using the BSC to integrate the organization's goals and values into everyday operations.[23] For instance, Russ and Susan Kershaw state, "The scorecard should guide the daily actions of the hospice unit staff to achieve the hospital's mission of providing patient-focused care."[24]

The application of institutional core values into individual decision making has been a touchstone of business ethics for more than a decade.[25] The involvement of organizational ethicists, and others interested in organizational ethics, in disseminating the values that are associated with the BSC recognizes that, especially in healthcare, as Terry Cooper writes, "real power is held by people at the various levels of an organization and not only by those at the top of the bureaucratic pyramid. Those with client interaction can distort or obstruct the organization's mission by the way services are delivered. . . ."[26]

The contribution of individuals committed to organizational ethics to communicating the values associated with the BSC may take many forms. A one-page memo can explicate the cause and effect between values and measures, directly connecting strategy to outcomes and the organization's mission.[27] Likewise, learning processes can be constructed to emphasize the organization's positive aspirations, rather than the negative connotations that typify the lay interpretation of "ethics."[28]

Since the perceived values of the organization help determine the ethical climate of the organization, disseminating the BSC and the values associated with it is entirely in keeping with the responsibility of organizational ethicists and others interested in organizational ethics to promote the positive ethical climate of the organization. Moreover, the involvement of ethicists in the evolution of a BSC would fulfill a repeated call for the integration of ethics committees into the overall organizational structure, with associated accountability for measurable organizational outcomes.[29] According to Ellen More, "Unquestionably, one test of a good health care organization is whether it encourages professionals to exercise sound, responsible judgment. . . ."[30] A properly constructed BSC in the hands of frontline associates who are well-trained in its application will lead to a level of consistency in service delivery yet to be seen in healthcare delivery organizations.

ONGOING MEASUREMENT AND ASSESSMENT

Changing or shifting the daily practices, values, or mission of an organization will require ongoing measurement and assessment.[31] Continuous monitoring of these measures keeps management in touch with the organization's performance and where it stands, right now, in the accomplishment of the organization's goals and values. In practice, this requires some internal communication mechanism (for example, intranet) that presents all measures in the scorecard, appropriate external comparison benchmarks, and real-time reporting in a single visual display.[32] But if organizations select and continuously monitor measures accurately and scientifically, major organizational disasters can be discovered and resolved before any material damage occurs.[33] Therefore, through contribution to determining the measures and methodology of the BSC and ensuring dissemination into daily practice, ethicists can help avert potentially catastrophic organizational ethical dilemmas.

Ethicists and others committed to maintaining a positive ethical climate may also serve an important role for re-evaluation of the measures used to ensure that values are not lost as performance improvement occurs. Paul Niven recommends assessing the BSC annually to check strategies against a changing environment, to test and retest measures, to survey internally to appraise employees' perception of the framework, and to plan for future development.[34] Organizational ethicists can take part in this review and ensure over time that the values and mission of the organization remain consistent within the BSC.

CHALLENGES FOR ACADEMIC MEDICAL CENTERS

Not all healthcare delivery organizations are alike. Unlike a typical community-based hospital, long-term care facility, or nonteaching hospital that focuses on their missions of patient care and community service, academic medical centers (AMCs) carry out the additional missions of research and teaching. The current competitive landscape threatens the traditional AMCs' missions and business model.[35] In this "for-profit era,"[36] distinctive components of the AMCs' mission have become endangered, as forces threaten its fundamental operating principles. AMCs are expected to provide state-of-the-art care to all, including private patients from professors' practice groups and clinic patients from local underserved populations. In addition, they are expected to care for the indigent.[37]

AMCs possess a unique set of structural characteristics that differentiate them from other teaching and nonteaching hospitals. For instance, members of the Association of American Medical Colleges Council of Teaching Hospitals provide clinical training for 75 percent of resident physicians in the U.S.[38]

Fusing the traditional hospital mission of patient care with the missions of clinical research, medical education, and service to poorer, severely ill, and clinically complex patients, necessitates an extremely complex, multifaceted organization, which Peter Drucker labels the most complex organization in history.[39] Achieving excellent function in this environment is a daunting task. Susan Mehrtens characterized AMCs as "plagued by inefficient operations, a bloated, slow-moving bureaucracy, complex organizational structures, and a complacency that prevents significant change."[40] In lieu of abandoning their social, research, or educational mission, AMCs have attempted to adapt to the competitive environment. Strategies that AMCs have adopted to survive include selling the AMC to larger for-profit systems,[41] horizontal integration,[42] and management and structural reforms.[43] These adaptive strategies have typically failed.[44] However, the AMCs' unique characteristics make the BSC management approach particularly appealing on multiple levels.

The complexity associated with the mission of the AMC in its operations manifests itself in a host of ways. For instance, the physician-patient interaction will often involve younger, less-experienced residents who approach patients with multiple agendas — learning or teaching new clinical skills as well as delivering high-quality care. As part of their skill competencies, internal medicine residents are expected to understand "systems-based practice" that integrates their daily practice into the larger organizational context.[45] BSC methods could potentially aid them in garnering a systems-level understanding and adjusting their practice to fit the organization's mission and values. Moreover, department chairs, often held to the fire on financial outcomes, may also find the BSC appealing as a way to move leadership's focus beyond finances into "bigger picture" considerations.[46] The BSC can also serve as the framework for developing and aligning strategic plans across every faculty members' clinical practice organization.[47] From the broadest perspective, leading management science, both in general[48] and specific to academic medical centers,[49] concurs that effective organizational change demands having a structure or framework in place before beginning to create or implement a specific performance improvement strategy.

THE BSC IN PRACTICE

A growing number of healthcare delivery organizations evaluate and manage performance using the BSC framework to decide between competing organizational interests in service of their overall missions.[50] A significant number of healthcare provider organizations have adopted the BSC framework: the Mayo Clinic,[51] Yale,[52] Henry Ford Health System,[53] St. Mary's Duluth,[54] Peel Memorial,[55] and many others.[56] Several healthcare provider organizations have advanced the integration of the BSC framework to a high degree of sophistication.

Three high-profile examples demonstrate the potential payoffs and pitfalls for those considering using the BSC: Duke University Hospital System, Baptist Health Care Corporation, and Robert Wood Johnson University Hospitals (RWJUH). These particular cases were selected for several reasons. Baptist Health Care Corporation and RWJUH represent the two most recent winners of the Malcolm Baldrige National Quality Award, a prestigious, non-industry-specific award for extraordinary quality that is rarely given to healthcare delivery organizations. Only four healthcare delivery organizations have received the honor in its 18-year history. Second, as health systems with academic medical centers, Duke and RWJUH model the BSC application in perhaps the most complex healthcare delivery organization setting possible. Finally, each encountered successes and difficulties that may be generalized to most healthcare delivery organizations.

DUKE UNIVERSITY HOSPITAL SYSTEM

Among the early adopters, Duke University Hospital System (DUHS) first began incorporating the BSC approach in 1996.[57] The first hospital system known to incorporate "internal business" with clinical quality, Duke spent significant time and energy at the beginning "setting the right structure, picking the right measures, and measuring the right way."[58] Duke's explicit goal was to create a cascading set of measures that had the ability to translate their strategic mission, vision, and values to the frontline.

In the well-publicized success story of Duke Children's Hospital (DCH), Jon Meliones, MD, commented on the implementation: "We explained the theory to clinicians and administrators like this: if you sacrifice too much in one quadrant to satisfy another, your organization as a whole is thrown out of balance.

We could, for example, cut costs to improve the financial quadrant by firing half the staff, but that would hurt quality of service, and the customer quadrant would fall out of balance...."[59] At Duke University's Birthing Center (DUBC), the BSC framework enabled clinicians and managers to envision tactics and goals that overlapped the key stakeholder perspectives of finance, customer, quality, and employee. Through the creation of a patient resource manager, improved physician services, streamlined patient flow, and the recruitment of innovative, multidisciplinary staff, DUBC achieved increased patient satisfaction, decreased length of stay, decreased costs, and, ultimately, improved the quality of service to women.[60]

To make the BSC a system-wide reality, DUHS established performance improvement teams for each quadrant of their BSC. The four quadrants are similar to the ones mentioned above, and included Clinical Quality and Internal Business, Customer Service, Work Culture, and Finances. Each quadrant is associated with a goal. For example, the goal associated with Clinical Quality and Internal Business is to foster enhanced clinical care and new program development, to improve quality, patient safety, and efficiency. The goal associated with Customer Service is to continuously improve customer service for both internal and external customers. The goal associated with Work Culture is to continuously improve the work culture, consistent with DUHS's values. The goal associated with Finances is to generate sufficient resources to reinvest in people, technology, buildings, research, and education. Steering these teams is a performance improvement oversight committee chaired by the system's chief executive officer (CEO). Real-time results are reviewed continuously by management while the BSC methodology is reviewed quarterly. Despite documented success, the goal of full assimilation throughout all areas of the organization has yet to be achieved. At year eight, DUHS reports reaching the department level, but has yet to fully execute the BSC down to the individual level.

To take the next step, DUHS is currently readjusting its compensation system to expressly link pay with performance. From executives to managers to frontline staff, each DUHS associate will have a set of specific measures and goals that support the overarching goals identified in the BSC. The DUHS human resources office states, "The power of the balanced scorecard lies in the linkage between these four perspectives. So, by improving the right organizational capabilities (Work Culture), you will improve your business processes (Clinical Quality and Internal Business), which result in improved customer perceptions (Customer Service), which in turn, lead to meeting your financial (Finances) objectives and achieving your vision."[61] It should also be noted that since the goals associated with the four perspectives reflect the values of DUHS, improving the organization's capabilities will go hand in hand with generating a shared ethical climate based on these values.

BAPTIST HEALTH CARE CORPORATION

The BSC approach originally delineated by CEO (then chief operating officer) Al Stubblefield, former Baptist Health Care administrator Quint Studer, and the rest of the management team, deliberately mirrored the mission and vision of their hospital: people, service, quality, growth, and finance.[62] These values were communicated as "pillars," forming the foundation of the organization. Planning for performance improvement strategies was based on them. Hence, the measurements used to assess improvement in departmental and individual decisions and outcomes were expressly tied with these pillars. Using this framework, Baptist Health Care Corporation achieved alignment with organizational values across service lines and down to the individual employee level.

Employees are introduced to the pillars even before filling out an application for employment. Each service line, department, unit, manager, and employee reports what they are doing to meet the goals or objectives under each pillar. The BSC, including its measures and results, are publicly communicated across the organization — on walls, bulletin boards, intranets, and newsletters. Every report, every meeting, every strategic plan, and every plan for improvement are structured around these values and measures. These organizational tactics result in a universal, clear understanding among all staff members of how what they do everyday contributes to the overarching organization's mission, vision, and values.

Aligning service excellence or clinical quality improvement project teams towards the same goals creates an opportunity to improve multiple outcomes simultaneously. In one case at Baptist Health Care, internal medicine physicians complained that too many patients got pressure ulcers during their hospital stay. After investigation, recognition of the problem, and communication with the medical staff, the team set about eliminating the problem. This involved several fronts: staff training, involving expert skilled nursing unit staff to transfer their best practices to other units, and tracking and publicly displaying the percentages of pressure ulcers on each unit. The overall rate dropped from 5 percent to 1.4 percent. It turned out that the unreimbursed cost of each pressure ulcer was on average $23,000, and patients with pressure ulcers gave far lower satisfaction ratings. Thus, in a single project, this one team improved medical staff satisfaction, clinical outcomes, patients' satisfaction, and reduced costs by several hundred thousand dollars.

ROBERT WOOD JOHNSON UNIVERSITY HOSPITALS

Robert Wood Johnson University Hospitals (RWJUH) (New Brunswick, New Jersey, and Hamilton, New Jersey) are the principal hospitals for the Robert Wood Johnson Medical School.[63] RWJUH created their BSC by first explicitly considering their stakeholder groups: employees, physicians, and the community. Similar to DUHS, RWJUH found that success in each area is highly related to success in the other — feeding either a virtuous or vicious cycle. When they began this strategy in 1998, RWJUH decided to spend equal time improving patient satisfaction, employee satisfaction, physician satisfaction, and the community's perceptions. RWJUH continually evaluated the measures and goals within each of these perspectives.

After defining their BSC and measures, RWJUH generated a weekly report card and dashboard with a traffic light indicator system (red, yellow, green) to intuitively indicate performance status. Red and yellow issues were identified for rapid analysis and action. RWJUH used qualitative data (patients' comments from surveys) to compile a complaint management database, trend the complaints over time, and take action to rectify the processes or people at the root cause. Physician-specific data is used to manage physicians' performance — which is exceptionally important in the emergency department (ED), where RWJUH provides an unparalleled service guarantee that all patients in the ED will be seen by a nurse within 15 minutes of arrival and will see a physician in 30 minutes — or the visit is free. RWJUH reduced the average ED waiting time for admission by 25 percent within three months, with a 60-minute wait time for ED admission into the hospital.

The same attention is devoted to employees' and physicians' satisfaction. The Employee Satisfaction Committee is an interdisciplinary team led by the CEO to identify opportunities for improvement. This group was influential in recommending enhancements to many policies and procedures, including employee wellness programs, healthy menus in the cafeteria, and a new "employee of the quarter" program. Handwritten notes are regularly sent to employees' homes recognizing acts of service excellence. Leaders are expected to round and identify positive behaviors. This easily implemented practice is received positively by employees. Employees receive bonuses based on patients' satisfaction results. Employees' satisfaction results show overall improvement to the 88th percentile. Most impressive were results in customer focus subscale (99th percentile), satisfaction with senior leadership (98th percentile), recognition subscale (91st percentile), and morale subscale (91st percentile). The hospital was recognized by the New Jersey Business and Industry Association as Best Employer related to this innovative process.

Indeed, RWJUH reports extraordinary results. RWJUH is among the fastest growing hospital systems in the Northeastern seaboard, with double-digit growth in volume and revenue every year over the past five years. From 1999 to 2003, emergency room visits swelled 100 percent, driving overall business up, with 70 percent of admissions coming through the emergency room. Market shares in cardiology, surgery, and oncology each grew at least 33 percent. The parent company, Robert Wood Johnson Health System, has transferred these methods to all seven of its acute-care hospitals.

DISCUSSION

Healthcare executives report several benefits from adopting the BSC approach. The development process forces executives to clarify and gain consensus on the organization's mission and values, and on strategies to achieve them. This increases senior management's credibility with board members, who can then more clearly understand the BSC's measures and results for which executives will be held accountable. After the BSC is developed, the values explicitly embedded in it give executives a framework for making decisions. A properly constructed BSC forces individuals' (including management) thinking and decision making to align with the organization's values. It also forces management to face any unpleasant facts that may be reported in the measurements. This helps executives set rational and appropriate priorities. In weighing multiple initiatives or projects, the BSC tightens the relationship between resource allocation and mission, vision, and values. Management accountability improves — especially when measures are linked to managers' incentive plans. Finally, continuous communication and communication of results encourages quality improvement initiatives, as the links between quality and financial returns become more obvious. [64]

The experiences reported here bear out the original purpose of the BSC: to achieve strategic clarity and improve executive decision making. Interested healthcare professionals and ethicists do not necessarily have to wait for senior leadership or the macro system to adopt a BSC management approach. The BSC works well at the micro-system level, as well. For example, it has been applied successfully in an academic clinical department,[65] a burn unit,[66] and public health clinics[67] without having the support of an overarching organizational BSC approach.

The imperative to produce results across a balanced set of nonfinancial measures has increased dramatically in the past several years. California insurers are already using pay-for-performance schemes for providers and hospitals.[68] Pay-for performance systems create immediate financial incentives for providers, reaching beyond making revenue dependent on the volume of patients. Leading the change is the Integrated Healthcare Association (IHA), a group of health plans, health systems, hospitals, medical group practices, leading academic experts, large employers/purchasers, and consumer representatives.[69]

Interest in pay-for-performance is increasing among all payers, particularly the federal government. Currently, Medicare has one demonstration project underway that provides reimbursement bonuses for the best-performing healthcare delivery organizations, according to a set of clinical quality measures.[70]

Policy experts expect this incentive system to be applied to the Centers for Medicare and Medicaid Services (CMS) Hospital Quality and HCAHPS (Hospital Consumer Assessment of Health Plans) initiatives. Observers predict that CMS will make the variable annual increase in Medicare reimbursement dependent upon both clinical quality and patients' satisfaction with the experience of care. Hospitals with the lowest ratings will be unlikely to receive their annual increase. As federal, state, and regional initiatives promote and incentivize performance under a balanced set of objectives,[71] will healthcare ethicists and others committed to organizational ethics play a role?

CONCLUSION

Organizational ethicists and others committed to a positive ethical climate have a substantial role to play in the development and adoption of a scorecard. In all three cases described above, the first step of organizational leaders was to identify the mission of the organization and articulate the values that would drive it. In all three cases, measures were identified so that the perspectives of legitimate stakeholders were ascertained and translated into goals that could be measured. In all three cases, communication of the BSC, its values, and its measures were essential to success, and in all three cases refinement of the BSC was seen as crucial to keeping the organization focused on what it wanted to achieve and how it would be achieved. Influencing the development of the BSC, actively seeking to communicate the values embedded in it, and being available to monitor and refine measures associated with outcomes should be seen as a responsibility of organizational ethicists, as the implementation of the BSC will affect the ethical climate of the organization, and that is the responsibility of organizational ethicists, together with others committed to organizational ethics. Just as healthcare professionals committed to creating a positive ethical climate will need new skills to be effective, organizational ethicists might have to acquire new skills to be effective, and it may be that some fear and intimidation is associated with acquiring these skills. But that is a small matter, compared with the appropriate evolution of their organization.

ACKNOWLEDGMENTS

The author acknowledges Kayhan Parsi, JD, PhD, of the Loyola University of Chicago Neiswanger Institute for Bioethics and Health Policy and Ann E. Mills of the Center for Biomedical Ethics at the University of Virginia Health System for their helpful reviews of this essay.

An earlier version of this chapter appeared in *Organizational Ethics: Healthcare, Business, and Policy*, volume 2, no.1 (Spring

2005). ©2005, University Publishing Group. Used with permission. All rights reserved.

NOTES

1. A.E. Mills, M.V. Rorty, and P.H. Werhane, "The Organization Ethics Process as a Vehicle for Change in Healthcare Delivery Organizations," *Organizational Ethics: Healthcare, Business, and Policy* 1, no. 1 (2004): 21-31.

2. R.R. Sims, "The challenge of ethical behavior in organizations," *Journal of Business Ethics* 11 (1992): 505-13.

3. C. Meyers, "Institutional culture and individual behavior: creating an ethical environment," *Science and Engineering Ethics* 10, no. 2 (April 2004): 269-76.

4. R. Hamel, "A question of value: What does ethics contribute to the life and work of an organization?" *Health Progress* 78, no. 3 (May-June 1997): 24-6, 32; J. Joseph and S.P. Deshpande, "The impact of ethical climate on job satisfaction of nurses," *Health Care Management Review* 22, no. 1 (Winter 1997): 76-81.

5. P.H. Werhane, "Organization Ethics, Systems Thinking, and Public/Private Partnerships in Health Care," (paper presented at the Loyola University-Chicago Conference on Organizational Ethics in Healthcare, 10-12 June 2004, Chicago, Ill.).

6. P.H. Werhane, "Business ethics, stakeholder theory, and the ethics of healthcare delivery organizations," *Cambridge Quarterly of Healthcare Ethics* 9 (2000): 169-181.

7. R.S. Kaplan and D.P. Norton, *The Balanced Scorecard: Translating Strategy into Action* (Boston, Mass.: Harvard Business School Press, 1996).

8. Werhane, see note 5 above.

9. R.S. Kaplan and D.P. Norton, "The balanced scorecard — measures that drive performance," *Harvard Business Review* 70, no. 1 (January-February 1992): 71-9.

10. R.S. Kaplan and D.P. Norton, *The Balanced Scorecard: Business: The Ultimate Resource* (Cambridge, Mass.: Perseus, 2002), 303-4, 510-11, 1001-11.

11. See note 7 above.

12. A.C. Maltz, A.J. Shenhar, R.R. Reilly, "Beyond the balanced scorecard: Refining the search for organizational success," *Long Range Planning* 36 (2003): 187-204.

13. C. Ells and C. MacDonald, "Implications of Organizational Ethics to Healthcare," *Healthcare Management Forum* 15, no. 3

(2002): 32-8; S.D. Pearson, J.E. Sabin, and E.J. Emanuel, *No Margin, No Mission: Health-Care Organizations and the Quest for Ethical Excellence* (London: Oxford University Press, 2003), 26.

14. S. Covey, *Principle-Centered Leadership* (New York: Free Press, 1992); F.J. Varela, *Ethical Know-How: Action, Wisdom, and Cognition* (Stanford, Calif.: Stanford University Press, 1992).

15. A. Weston, *A Practical Companion to Ethics* (London: Oxford University Press, 1997).

16. L. Randel et al., "How managed care can be ethical," *Health Affairs* 20, no. 4 (July-August 2001): 43-56.

17. D.F. Thompson, "The possibility of administrative ethics," *Public Administration Review* 45 (1985): 555-61.

18. M.K. Wynia, "Performance measures for ethics quality," *Effective Clinical Practice* 2 (1999): 294-99.

19. J.W. Cartwright, S.C. Stolp-Smith, and E. Edell, "Strategic performance management: Development of a performance measurement system at Mayo Clinic," *Journal of Healthcare Management* 45, no. 1 (2000): 58-68.

20. G.H. Pink, "Creating a balanced scorecard for a hospital system," *Journal of Health Care Finance* 27, no. 3 (2001): 1-20.

21. M.B. Rosenthal et al., "Paying for quality: Providers' incentives for quality improvement," *Health Affairs* 23, no. 2 (2004): 127-41.

22. C.R. Denham, "The no-outcome, no-income tsunami: Surviving 'pay 4 performance'," *Focus on Patient Safety* 7, no. 1(2004):1-3; *http://www.npsf.org/download/Focus 004vol7No1.pdf.*

23. B.E. Becker, M.A. Huselid, and D. Ulrich, *The HR Scorecard: Linking People, Strategy, and Performance* (Boston, Mass.: Harvard Business School Press, 2001).

24. R. Kershaw and S. Kershaw, "Developing a balanced scorecard to implement strategy at St. Elsewhere Hospital," *Management Accounting Quarterly* (Winter 2001) online journal, *http://www.imanet.org/ima/sec.asp?TRACKID=&CID=860&DID=1167*; M.L. Jones, "Strategy management system in perinatal services: the role of a patient resource manager," *Lippincott's Case Management* 7, no. 1 (2002): 27-42, *http://www.nursing center.com/prodev/ce_article.asp?tid= 260642,* accessed 27 June 2004.

25. P.J. Dean, "Making codes of ethics real," *Journal of Business Ethics* 9 (1992): 285-90.

26. T.L. Cooper, *The Responsible Administrator: An Approach*

to *Ethics for the Administrative Role* (San Francisco, Calif.: Jossey-Bass, 1998), 180.

27. R.S. Kaplan and D.P. Norton, *The Strategy Focused Organization* (Boston, Mass.: Harvard Business School Press, 2001).

28. D.T. Ozar, "The gold standard for ethics education and effective decision making in healthcare delivery organizations," *Organizational Ethics: Healthcare, Business, and Policy* 1, no. 1 (2004): 32-42.

29. D.C. Blake, "Organizational ethics: Creating structural and cultural change in healthcare delivery organizations," *The Journal of Clinical Ethics* 10, no. 2 (Summer 1999): 187-93.

30. E.S. More, "The remains of the profession, or what the butler knew," *Annals of Internal Medicine* 134, no. 3 (2001): 255-9.

31. M. Van Wart, "The First Step in the Reinvention Process: Assessment" in *The Ethics Edge,* ed. E.M. Berman, J.P. West, and S.J. Bonczek (Washington, D.C.: International City/County Management Association, 1998): 80-100.

32. J. Wyatt, "Scorecards, dashboards, and KPIs: Keys to integrated performance measurement," *Healthcare Financial Management* (February 2004): 76-80.

33. K.G. McGee, *Heads Up: How to Anticipate Business Surprises and Seize Opportunities First* (Boston, Mass.: Harvard Business School Press, 2004).

34. P.R. Niven, *Balanced Scorecard Step-by-Step: Maximizing Performance and Maintaining Results* (New York: John Wiley & Sons, 2002).

35. D. Blumenthal, E.G. Campbell, and J.S. Weissman, "The social missions of academic health centers," *New England Journal of Medicine* 337 (1997): 1550-3.

36. Association of American Medical Colleges, "Teaching Hospitals," *http://www. aamc.org/teachinghospitals.htm,* accessed 23 December 2004.

37. See note 35 above.

38. See note 36 above.

39. From a seminar presented by Peter F. Drucker on 27 September 2003, "What Are the Results of Measuring Corporate Performance?" *http://www.projectauditors.com/Papers/Whiteppprs/Drucker092703.pdf,* accessed 22 April 2004.

40. S.E. Mehrtens, "The law of the retarding lead," *Perspectives on Business & Global Change* 14, no. 2 (June 2000): 12-5.

41. See note 19 above.
42. B.W. Harber, "The balanced scorecard at Peel Memorial Hospital," *Hospital Quarterly* 1, no. 4 (1998): 59-63.
43. E.W. Strenger, "The data game: Play it right, and you could win more managed care contracts," *Trustee* 50, no. 4 (1997): 7-11, 28.
44. E.A. Kazemek, P.R. Knecht, and B.G. Westfall, "Effective boards: Working smarter to meet the challenge," *Trustee* 53, no. 5 (2000): 18-24.
45. American Osteopathic Association and American College of Osteopathic Internists, *Basic Standards for Residency Training in Internal Medicine* (July 2004), http://www.acoi.org/BasicStandards.pdf, accessed 1 January 2005.
46. D.P. Tarantino, "Using the Balanced Scorecard as a performance management tool — nuts and bolts of business," *Physician Executive* 29, no. 5 (September-October 2003): 69-72.
47. S. Rimar, "Strategic planning and the balanced scorecard for faculty practice plans," *Academic Medicine* 75, no. 12 (2000): 1186-8.
48. R.S. Kaplan and D.P. Norton, "Linking the balanced scorecard to strategy," *California Management Review* 39, no. 1 (1996): 53-79; J. Collins, *Good to Great: Why Some Companies Make the Leap . . . and Others Don't* (New York: HarperBusiness, 2001).
49. T. Gilmore, L. Hirschhorn, and M. Kelly, *Challenges of leading and planning academic medical centers* (white paper), (Philadelphia, Penn.: Center for Applied Research, 1999), http://www.cfar.com/pdf/acdmdctr.pdf, accessed 1 January 2005.
50. J.R. Griffith, *Designing 21st Century Healthcare: Leadership in Hospitals and Healthcare Systems* (Chicago, Ill.: Health Administration Press, 1998).
51. See note 19 above.
52. See note 42 above.
53. See note 43 above.
54. See note 44 above.
55. See note 47 above.
56. K.E. Voelker, J.S. Rakich, and G.R. French, "The balanced scorecard in healthcare delivery organizations: a performance measurement and strategic planning methodology," *Hospital Topics* 79, no. 3 (2001): 13-24; W.N. Zelman et al., "Issues for academic health centers to consider before implementing a balanced-scorecard effort," *Academic Medicine* 74, no. 12 (1999): 1269-77.

57. G. Shulby, "Evolution to Revolution: A Journey Towards Excellence," in *Quantifying Health Care: Blueprint* (Durham, N.C.: American College of Healthcare Executives, 15 June 2004).

58. Ibid.

59. J. Meliones, "Saving money, saving lives," *Harvard Business Review* 78, no. 6 (2000): 57-62, 64, 66-7.

60. Jones, see note 60 above.

61. *http://www.hr.duke.edu/payperformance/achieving_ our_goals/balanced_ scorecard.html,* accessed 1 January 2005.

62. A. Stubblefield, *The Baptist Health Care Journey to Excellence: Creating a Culture* (New York: John Wiley & Sons, 2004).

63. *Malcolm Baldrige National Quality Award 2004 Award Recipient, Health Care: Robert Wood Johnson University Hospital Hamilton,* 2004, *http://www.nist.gov/public_affairs/releases/ rwj_hamilton.htm,* accessed 27 June 2004

64. N. Inamdar and Kaplan, "Applying the balanced scorecard in healthcare provider organizations," *Journal of Healthcare Management* 47, no. 3 (2002): 179-95.

65. See note 47 above.

66. I.L. Wachtel, C.E. Hartford, and J.A. Hughes, "Building a balanced scorecard for a burn center," *Burns* 25, no. 5 (1999): 431-7.

67. V.A. Robinson, D. Hunter, and S.E. Shortt, "Accountability in public health units: using a modified nominal group technique to develop a balanced scorecard for performance measurement," *Canadian Journal of Public Health* 94, no. 5 (2003): 391-6.

68. M.E. Lanser, "Pay-for-Performance in California: The IHA Model," *Healthcare Executive* (March/April 2005): 26-7.

69. Ibid.

70. For details, see: *http://www. cms. hhs.gov/quality/* and *http://www.cms.hhs. gov/researchers/demos/phqi/default.asp.*

71. T.J. Hill, "Hospital performance improvement and the balanced scorecard," *Satisfaction Monitor* (May/June 2004): 1-4.

The Financial Perspective

4

Professionalism in Medicine and in Business

Lisa H. Newton

INTRODUCTION

Both physicians and business managers think of themselves as "professionals." In what does their professionalism consist? And are their professionalisms compatible? The question is raised with particular urgency by the ACGME's (Accreditation Council for Graduate Medical Education) call for medical residents in hospitals, whose education the ACGME guides, to "demonstrate a commitment to ethical principles pertaining to provision or withholding of clinical care, confidentiality of patient information, informed consent, and business practices."[1] Later in the ACGME guidelines, under "systems-based practice," residents are expected to understand "methods of controlling health care costs and allocating resources," and to "practice cost-effective health care and resource allocation that does not compromise quality of care." That last is a tall order. Subsequent guidelines emphasize the importance of physicians knowing "how to partner with health care managers and health care providers to assess, coordinate, and improve health care." Are such partnerships possible? Are they good?

In this chapter we will examine the roots of the professional ethics of physicians and business managers, to bring forth, first, a clear and robust (non-straw) portrait of the professional in both fields; second, and of primary importance to this chapter, to indicate the patent areas of incompatibility, and to draw out the implications of that incompatibility for professional integrity; and third, we shall try to find areas where organizational ethics, the ethics of the business organizations that manage healthcare, can resolve the problems raised in the previous sections.

TWO, OR RATHER THREE, ETHICAL COMMITMENTS

In the course of teaching medical ethics (or healthcare ethics), we always begin with the "professional commitment of the physician." That ethic, hereinafter PCP, is derived from the old "medical ethic," descended from the Hippocratic Oath. The traditional form of the Oath, as you will recall, begins by invoking Apollo Physician and a host of minor deities, goes on to make a series of impractical (and occasionally illegal) promises of financial support to the physician's teacher and the teacher's family, continues with a series of medical standards and specific prohibitions — good dietary advice, no euthanasia, no abortion, no surgery, no practice whatsoever except for the benefit of the sick person, no sex with patients or the patients' household — and concludes with a promise of confidentiality on all matters relating to the patient and his treatment.

Many medical schools still require this Oath of all graduating students. The Oath in this form is clearly one among many pagan medical ethics. Ludwig Edelstein analyzes it as the product of a Pythagorean brotherhood,[2] whose views on the sacredness of life and blood would have accounted for its prohibitions of abortion and surgery, which were not typical of the time; a treatise on surgery is found in the Hippocratic corpus,[3] and Aristotle routinely prescribes abortion in cases where a pregnancy is ill-timed or otherwise undesirable.[4]

In this form, obviously, the Oath does not seem to capture any consensus on the obligations of the ancient physician, let alone the contemporary physician. Yet no one is quite willing to throw it away: when pressures of time or temptations assault the physician, there needs to be some foundation for the plain duty to care for the patient, according to one's best medical judgment, to the exclusion of other considerations, found in paragraphs three and seven in the Oath. For this reason, Louis Lasagna (from Tufts Medical School) developed an updated form of the Oath in 1964. This version subtracts the gods and the promises to the teachers, and introduces some new considerations, a respect for the scientific basis of medicine, a recognition of the art that complements the science, and compassion — the acceptance of the patient as a full human being (not a "case"), and a felt obligation to care for that patient. Retained is the commitment to practice medicine only for the welfare of the patient, in accordance with the best medical knowledge.[5]

The moral basis for the PCP is the patient in the bed — frightened, disabled, often confused and in pain; in short, helpless. In that state, patients should be able to assume, face to face with the physician at the bedside, that this person is interested in healing them, and in nothing else. Even considerations of allocation of resources, justice, or desert — the social worth of the patient, the relative need of other patients, the cost of treatments — does not enter into the relationship between the physician and the patient. In an odd sort of way, considerations of justice are contaminants in the physician-patient relationship, distracting the physician's attention from the needs of this patient here and now.

The Anglo-American Common Law has a place for the PCP, in the ancient legal category of Fiduciary Obligation. When a legal contract is necessary between two parties of radically unequal power and knowledge — between parent and child, for instance, or between the manager of a complicated financial trust and its beneficiaries — the law imposes on the more knowledgeable and powerful party an obligation of faith, *fides*, that any action taken by that party shall be only for the benefit of the weaker party, the beneficiary. In law, that fiduciary obligation exists between all professionals and their clients — between physician and patient, lawyer and client, teacher and student. The PCP does not fit easily in the fiduciary obligation slot, which requires that the fiduciary be able to demonstrate before a judge, at regularly scheduled intervals, that every transaction executed by the trust, for instance, advanced the financial interests of the beneficiary.

Nothing in healthcare is that easy to demonstrate, and, eventually, every medical measure fails and the patient dies. But the existence of that obligation surely means that the law will back up the physician's decision to provide beneficial treatment for any patient with whom he or she has a professional-client relationship, that is, any patient in his or her practice. The law will also listen seriously to any patient's legal challenge to the effect that the physician abused that trust, by malpractice, that is, practicing medicine negligently (lacking the appropriate knowledge or failing to employ the accepted beneficial measures to heal the patient), or by abandoning the patient. Not every challenge will succeed; a jury will have to decide whether the plaintiff or the defendant will prevail in a malpractice suit. But if the patient can produce evidence that the physician in this case had good reason to maltreat or to abandon his or her patients, the jury will not think kindly of the physician. Malpractice suits loom large in the practice of medicine (one reason that tort reform is always on the political agenda), so this point is worth remembering.

The PCP, the physician-patient obligation, is the first of the three ethics we have in conflict. The second is the free enterprise market commitment, hereinafter FEMC, which governs the businessperson in the marketplace. Derived from the proof of the superiority of free markets to government regulation in Adam Smith's *Wealth of Nations*,[6] the FEMC requires every participant in the market to seek his own interest first and last, and leave "the common good" to the work of the "Invisible Hand," which inevitably rewards efficiency and therefore brings about the greatest good for the greatest number.

The system demands that some tradesmen and merchants, the more efficient, who can bring their goods to market at the lowest cost and the highest quality, succeed, while others, the less efficient, fail and go out of business. The successful player in the market is not absolutely required to gloat and brag over his success, but pity or compassion for his less successful competitor in the market, to the point where he modifies his prices or choice of goods in trade in order to leave room for him, is forbidden. For the good of all, the market must be allowed free rein to sort the good from the bad, and the result of the sorting will be the most possible goods available, at the best possible quality and price, for all consumers. This freedom is not a license to steal. Indeed, the free market depends on a set of fixed moral rules, including absolute honesty (in representation of goods), respect for private property, transparency in all agreements, and the absolute sanctity of contract — no man may sign a contract because it is in his interest to sign it, then refuse to perform it because it is not in his interest to perform! Merchants may, of course, out of Christian duty or a shrewd perception of the opinions of their neighbors, decide to give away some of their profit to help the poor, but charity is strictly a personal choice.

In this system, oddly, compassion is a contaminant, mirroring the position of justice as a contaminant in the physician-patient relationship. Compassion, here, often serves as a motive for ill-advised governmental interference in the generally beneficent operations of the market.

Of course the businessperson does not have to run every aspect of her business herself. She can delegate parts of it to others, with instructions as to how they are to do the job in order to further the interests of the business. If the delegate works directly under her supervision, as an employee, he can be expected to do nothing other than what he is told, and it is the employer's responsibility, as owner of the business, to make sure that the employee's actions further the interests of the business. But if the business is complex, a modern corporation with advanced technology spread over several continents, she may hire a person with special expertise to attend to a portion of the complexities, with no instructions other than "to use your expertise to further the interests of the corporation." In that case, a different relationship is set up between the woman and the employee — she becomes the "principal," the person for whom all action is performed, and the expert employee becomes an "agent" of that principal with the responsibility of serving the principal's interests.

The relationship that governs principal and agent is the same as that governing physician and patient: the principal is the beneficiary, the agent is the fiduciary, and the relationship is one of fiduciary obligation. The agent may not (in his official capacity) do anything that is not for the benefit of the principal. In that modern corporation, of course, the "employer" would probably not be a single woman, but millions of shareholders, spread over as many continents as the business itself. The corporation itself, the fictional person administered by a board of directors, fiduciary for all the shareholders, is the principal in the relationship. The managers of the corporation are agents of that principal, and as managers, are committed to serve it; we may call this the professional commitment of the manager, or PCM.

The duties involved in a fiduciary relationship, as above, are quite clear. The fiduciary must serve the interests of the beneficiary. Professional managers must manage the company in the interests of the shareholders, that is, to increase the value of their stock in the company. (The shareholders have many interests beside financial — spiritual, emotional, and aesthetic, for instance

— but the corporate managers are charged only with the financial end of their lives.) They may be tempted to do other things with the money they manage than use it to make more money — they might, for instance, be tempted to contribute to a local opera company or a settlement house for the poor. But they cannot do this, unless they are prepared to demonstrate that in the short to medium run (no one is in the market for the long run any more) the increase in community good will purchased by these contributions will materially aid the fortunes of the corporation. After all, it isn't *their* money. In the logic of the relationship, here as above, compassion for the suffering and civic spirit in support of community enterprises, so admirable in the individual life of the citizen, are contaminants in the activity of pursuing the interests of the corporation, temptations that the manager must (logically) resist. Corporations regularly do exhibit civic spirit, of course, but that's because, thank goodness, the system does not operate strictly according to its internal logic. (The American public may want to ask, eventually, if we should correct the system at its logical root or count on its continuing to operate flexibly.)

The relationship that will be of special interest to this chapter is that created when a physician is hired by an insurance company or health-maintenance organization, a business whose business is healthcare. We expect that the business will be carried on in an ethical manner, that is, in a professional manner. We expect that the professionals involved in the enterprise will be aware of their obligations and will carry them out fully and faithfully. By this point in the game, what obligations are we talking about?

There are three ethics, or linked sets of obligations, on the table: (1) PCP, the professional obligation of the physician (or other healthcare provider) to attend only to the individual patient, and to use the full panoply of medical expertise available to help that patient to regain health; (2) FEMC, the right and duty of the business enterprise in the free market system to use any legal means to increase profits, without regard to any long-range "general good" or concern for the suffering of individuals; and (3) PCM, the fiduciary obligation of the professional manager to serve the financial interests of the shareholders. How might these three sets of obligations interact, especially for the physician, in the managed-care society?

RECIPES FOR CATASTROPHE

There are times when a page of history is worth a volume of logic. The perspective of this chapter is that of the professional, who, in attempting to honor the obligations that attend his profession and his employment, discovers that there are conflicts. Another possible perspective is that of the consumer, the patient as consumer of medical care, the physician as consumer of fees, the country as a whole as consumer of the healthcare system. How on earth did everyone's expectations get so high, that there is so much discontent floating around in the system? One of the reasons we find it so difficult to cope with our current healthcare system is that we got used to a particularly beneficent nonsystem in the past half century. About midcentury, a substantial portion of the citizenry abandoned the traditional family model of healthcare, in which all coping and curing took place in the home, and adopted the medical model, centered now in the high-tech hospital. Birth and death for the first time now (generally) took place in that hospital, physicians made all decisions, and a miraculous web of healthcare insurance, extending over most of the employed, reimbursing physicians at their usual rates, supplemented our traditional philanthropy-supported nonprofit hospitals. It doesn't take long to get used to medical miracles supplied at low or no cost. This particular idyll ended when the proliferation of technology, encouraged by the promise of a good return on investment, drove healthcare costs beyond what anyone had envisioned. In 1993, the year that William Jefferson Clinton took office as President of the United States, total healthcare expenditures in the United States stood at $888.1 billion, or 13.4 percent of the U.S. gross domestic product (GDP).[7] That was considered to be much too high; it was certainly higher than any other developed nation spends for healthcare. Something had to be done.

Our most recent opportunity to do something culminated in a national debate (1992-1994) on the possibility of a nationalized healthcare plan. Clinton had been elected to the presidency on the promise of making good healthcare universally available. In 1992, when the debate over the Clinton Plan began, the objective of lowering costs had assumed first priority. When the plan was finally voted down, healthcare expenditures were still going up; by 1995, they were up to $988.5 billion, or 13.6 percent of the U.S. GDP.[8] With the Clinton Plan no longer an option, the arrangement adopted by much of the country was to extend the reach of private insurance plans, many of which had been in place for several decades, and to create the new class of managed-care organizations (MCOs), (or health-maintenance organizations — HMOs), in which subscribers could arrange for future healthcare needs through prepayment for standard plans.[9] These rapidly spread to include a substantial portion of the population. While the wealthiest of Americans continue to pay privately for their own healthcare, and most (but not all) of the poorest Americans continue to subsist on state-administered Medicaid, the majority of those in between are covered, more or less, by this private insurance system. (Medicare is divided between a straight federal government system and one filtered through HMOs).[10] In the course of the national discussion of the Clinton Plan, it became clear that, as a citizenry, we were on the horns of a trilemma. A "dilemma," as we know, is a set of two sentences, both of which cannot be true. A "trilemma" is a set of three sentences, any two of which can be true, but not all three of which can be true. As used in policy debates, the trilemma tends to denote a set of three desiderata, desirable states, any two of which are attainable, but all three of which cannot simultaneously obtain. In the case of healthcare, the desirable states were well-known. We want:

1. The highest quality of medical care available anywhere in the world;
2. Universal access to that care, regardless of ability to pay;
3. As a percentage of the GDP, low and stable costs for that care.

We can have (1) and (2), but the costs will be through the roof; (2) and (3), but the healthcare will be bargain-basement crude (*vide*: the Soviet system, through most of its history); (1) and (3), but everyone will have to pay cash, and most of the poor will not be cared for at all. Of course, the American consumer of healthcare internalizes all those desiderata at different points of his interaction with the healthcare system: (3) when he selects his insurance plan, he looks only at costs, accepting all sorts of limits to access and advanced interventions, because right now he's healthy and he wants as much of his paycheck as he can get for disposable income; (2) when he gets sick, he wants access now, to any part of the system; (1) when he's being prepped for surgery, he wants the best surgeon and the most advanced techniques in the country. The trilemma lives in all of us, and a problem of legitimacy arises in any system that cannot bind them in one — that does not restore integrity to the patient, and to the physician-patient relationship, at the point of treatment.

Let us consider the MCO, the organization that now runs healthcare. There are many varieties of these organizations, too many to analyze separately. We will take one kind as emblematic of the others, for the same ethical problems arise in all of them. The emblematic MCO is an insurance company, that sells healthcare to individuals and to corporations that provide healthcare benefits for their employees. The MCO then hires physicians, nurses, and other healthcare providers to serve their insureds. (A more common arrangement has the MCO contract with a series of specialty practices — neurologists, ophthalmologists, primary care specialists — and treat the whole medical group as if it were an individual.)

There is nothing wrong with these organizations. There is a demand in the market for healthcare, indeed a demand that grows by the day. There are professionals, doctors and nurses, trained to service that demand, so the company hires them to provide that service. There is nothing unusual about "hiring professionals." Every corporation has professional accountants on staff, and any corporation involved in manufacturing complex technology hires trained engineers. Physicians and nurses can certainly be hired to practice medicine and nursing. To be sure, the American Medical Association (AMA) objected to these corporations, as having the potential to interfere in the free exercise of medical judgment, and affect the PCP. From the point of view of the free market, all such objections, and the rules that followed from them (no advertising; no ownership of medical facilities, et cetera) were just so many restrictions on free market and free trade. In the resulting confrontation, the restrictions lost — they are gone, probably forever.

Once the new organizations were in place, new management problems were discovered. Unlike engineers and accountants, physicians had not been socialized with the expectation of being loyal employees, agents of the employer. They expected to make their own decisions without consulting with their supervisors, no matter what the cost of those decisions might be to the employer. Reminding physicians of their obligations to increase efficiency by keeping down the costs to the business apparently did little good. The problem, as widely diagnosed (especially in the business theory literature on "agency theory"), is called "moral hazard": any situation in which the person or persons making an economically consequential choice bears no economic consequences for the choice carries with it the chance that the chooser(s) will not make the most responsible, or efficient, choice available in the situation. (For instance, if we allow the head of the marketing department to choose her office furniture without any budget to consider, she'll probably fill the room with French Provincial antiques. Better choices are available.) Physicians, in concert with their patients, were making all the choices on medical treatments, referrals, and pharmaceuticals, completely without regard to the cost, since neither had to bear that cost.

The insurance companies had no choice but to make patients and physicians share part of the risk that was covered by the healthcare plans. Accordingly, insurance contracts increasingly included "co-pay" provisions for the insured, requiring a payment of $5 to $25 at time of treatment, not enough to deter anyone who was truly sick, but enough to deter the "worried well," the employees who would visit physicians just because they didn't feel just right — and why not? It was already paid for.

Similarly, the contracts signed with the physicians increasingly included provisions for "hold-backs" and "bonuses": a physician who, in the course of the year, prescribed more than a certain average of expensive tests or brand-name drugs (with no permission to substitute less expensive generic varieties), or generated more than the average referrals to expensive specialists, might have some of his reimbursement "held back" at the end of the year; a physician who, on the contrary, held such tests, prescriptions, and referrals in check might expect a pleasant end-of-year bonus, just like the nonmedical executives in the administrative suites. A true "outlier," a physician who prescribed and referred at such a high level as to stand out in the cost counting at the end of the year, might find herself "de-selected," that is, barred from attending any of the insureds of that company.

De-selection amounts, in this case, to getting fired; the physician's practice is simply gone, leaving her no choice but to relocate and attempt to establish practice somewhere else. For a young professional with family, mortgage, and an average of $250,000 in student loans to repay, that possibility may be devastating. The contracts went beyond rewards and punishments, often specifying the content of the physician-patient encounter.

For instance, no patient would want to hear that a treatment or medication was available for her condition, but that, unfortunately, her insurance contract didn't cover it, so it could not be offered (with indication, if requested, of precisely where in the contract it was ruled out). So physicians were strongly counseled not to mention such treatments; these provisions in the contract were widely known as "gag orders."

Objections to all such contracts were raised immediately on behalf of the PCP. The physician was supposed, we recall, to have nothing at all of self-interest between her and her patient. She was supposed to stand at the bedside, or in the examining room, with nothing but the patient's benefit on her mind, and was supposed to summon all her knowledge to advise the patient (on diet and medication), to treat the patient using all her skill, and to stand aside for those more expert in the field (for example, refer to specialists) whenever the patient's condition required it. But she had no choice about signing the contracts. In many parts of the country, the entire healthcare industry is dominated by giant insurance companies, whose policies cover all potential patients who are covered at all. The individual physician who does not sign will have no patients. And if the physicians collectively refuse to sign a contract repugnant to their Oath, they are likely to find themselves in court sued by the insurance companies for conspiracy in restraint of trade.

The complaints of the physicians at the onerous demands of these contracts — especially in consideration of the obvious conflict of interest created by those "hold-back" clauses, which would have destroyed the chances of any physician to a fair trial in any malpractice proceedings — did not go unheard in state legislatures. By now, most states have outlawed those provisions that force physicians into direct conflict with their patients. This pattern is relatively new, and worth noting: in pursuit of competitive advantage, as required by PCM, the MCOs write rule after rule that lowers costs by (apparently) lowering service to patients. Patients and physicians raise a lugubrious howl. The sympathetic legislature acts, and the burdensome provision is now removed, with bad tastes all around: first, the legislative provision is of necessity a one-size-fits-all, and cannot be individualized as medicine individualizes; second, in the public mind, the insurance company is cast as something with horns and a tail; third, everyone now knows that another provision, just as heartless, might come along at any moment, so legislative supervision of healthcare, a very expensive proposition, rapidly expands to guard against it.[11]

Once the all-encompassing contract is signed, there is nothing to stop the insurance company from renegotiating that contract every year, lowering reimbursement each time.[12] The physician has the choice of relocating (but MCO-free areas in which to practice are getting harder to find), declaring bankruptcy (which has, at least, the prospect of release from the $250,000 debt left over from medical school), or moonlighting in the emergency room of the local hospital to supplement his specialty income.

How far can this system go? The business managers are not cruel, they are just under a mandate to increase profits each year. If they can do that by expanding their market, they will. If they can raise prices to their customers, the major corporations that buy their policies for their employees, they will do that. If they can find increased efficiencies in office procedures, they will cut costs by realizing those efficiencies. But the markets are crowded, and the competition for customers is fierce, and, with new regulations, it's tough to pare the office staff. If the only way to increase the profit is to lower reimbursements for the physicians, and their customers do not object, that is what the company will have to do. So the tendency is to lower reimbursements, year after year, as far as the traffic will bear — that is, until the physicians, or the medical practices, cannot make a living at that level of reimbursement, and refuse to sign the contract. The market works as it has always worked: the more efficient providers will stay in business, while the less efficient do not. Possibly some of the more efficient providers will hire some of the physicians in the failed practices, and teach them more efficient ways.

A troubling objection arises at this point. That analysis treats medical care like a giant Wal-Mart, where the customers prefer to do their shopping because the products are so inexpensive. Thoughtful shoppers will consider why the goods are so inexpensive, considering the conditions under which they are made, worrying about the nutritional status of the poor Southeast Asian worker who assembled the radio, saddened by the tales of underpaid non-union employees at Wal-Mart, genuinely regretting the human and environmental damage done in order to keep the prices so low. (*Very* thoughtful shoppers may not shop at Wal-Mart.) But it will never occur to any shopper that possibly the goods being purchased are of lower quality, maybe dangerously lower quality, just because of the compensation plans for the various levels of employees. Here's where the professions as a whole, and medicine in particular, are different from retailing.

Ultimately, the patient's healthcare dollar purchases the services of a physician. That much has not changed since Hippocrates. What has changed is the number of sticky fingers in between the patient and the physician, taking little pieces out of the dollar until there is little left for the physician. Physicians, like Wal-Mart's maintenance workers, will try to maintain their income in the face of lowering reimbursement by extending their hours or working more quickly. But a physician tired from working all night in an emergency room, or committed to dismissing patients after only four minutes of consultation in order to increase billable units, is very likely to lower the quality of her service — to miss asking the crucial questions, to fail to give that extra reassurance that will convince the patient to take the medication, to omit the follow up that would make sure the medicine is working as it should. And the real danger is that neither the consumer (the trusting patient in the waiting room) nor the customer (the human resources departments of the corporations that employ the patient) will know the difference. The physician might recognize the difference and regret it, but she probably feels she has no choice in the matter, and no one else is in a position to check up. It will be only after years of less-than-optimum practice that a pattern of worse-than-expected outcomes would be noticed by anyone outside the profession; given the inherent uncertainties of health, small variations would probably mean nothing at all.

What if the physician cannot bring himself to cut back systematically on the quality of the patient's care? What if he wants to refer a patient to a specialist, or order tests that he thinks will serve the patient's welfare, but that will not be reimbursable under the patient's insurance plan, given the patient's current condition or symptoms? Can he just lie to the insurance company about the patient's symptoms, so the referral or tests will become reimbursable? It has never been our custom to ask this question about a profession whose Hippocratic Oath includes, "In purity and holiness I will guard my life and my art." But given the clash of professional obligations documented here, it will come as no surprise that the question is alive, well, and living in Philadelphia: according to a recent report in the *American Jour-*

nal of Bioethics, up to half of Philadelphia residents turn out, under certain conditions, to support physicians' deceptive representation of patients' symptoms to secure reimbursement for tests and referrals.[13] The sentiment is not surprising; we have known for some time that some physicians gladly manipulate the rules of the system to help their patients.[14] Yet can lying and cheating be justified? Opinion is divided: in the comments following that report, one author notes the "deontological double jeopardy" in which physicians are placed by the conflict of fiduciary obligations,[15] others are clear that we must go "back to basics" in ethics — do not lie, cheat, or steal (noting that "gaming the system" to increase reimbursements is a case of all three, not to mention illegal.)[16] This position has been best (at least most forcefully) argued by Haavi Morreim, in *Balancing Act* (1995).[17]

What has happened, that a significant portion of physicians and patients now seem to expect physicians to (in effect) lie, cheat, and steal to fulfill their traditional obligation to protect the patient from all harm and injustice? That obligation is under very untraditional pressure, and the professional medical ethic, clear as glass a half a century ago, may be under this cloud for the rest of this generation.

What might the future hold for this set of professional ethical dilemmas? First, it may be noted that the HMO experiment has not lowered healthcare costs; by 2002, they stood at $1,559 billion in the U.S., or 14.9 percent of the GDP; the 2004 projection is $1,804.7 billion, or 15.4 percent of the GDP, and they are projected to hit $3,585.7 billion by 2014, or 18.7 percent of GDP.[18] That's very high. The problem is not going to go away by itself.

Second, it should be acknowledged that the poisonous conflicts outlined in this chapter are not inevitable, and that the emergence of a new organizational ethic begins to hold out hope of reconciliation. It is possible to run a healthcare system without the business or administrative end of it placing grinding pressures on the medical end, while the medical folks retaliate with falsified claims and invented symptoms. But the ethic that guides the healthcare organization, the organizational ethic, has to be ultimately respectful of the practice of medicine and the demands placed on the physician by the original medical ethic, or it will not work. It is doubtful indeed that the profit-oriented private sector, especially in its present investor-driven form, will provide institutions that are capable of disinterested management of healthcare. It is even more doubtful that government monitoring of that private sector, intervening in medical practice and HMO rules with one-size-fits-all protective legislation, will remedy the matter effectively. We look for the emergence of a new quasi-public institution, on the model perhaps of the National Oceanic and Atmospheric Agency (NOAA), which carries on its scientific work quietly and unmolested on public funds, yet can respond to the changing needs of an increasingly medically sophisticated population. More research is needed on the type of institutional arrangements that will be adequate to meet the varied needs of the healthcare system in the remainder of the century.

ACKNOWLEDGMENT

A version of the first part of this chapter will appear (toward a different end) in *The Ethics of Bioethics: Examining the Moral Landscape,* edited by Lisa Eckenwiler and Felicia Cohn. An earlier version appeared in *Organizational Ethics: Healthcare, Business, and Policy*, volume 2, no.1 (Spring 2005). ©2005, University Publishing Group. Used with permission. All rights reserved.

NOTES

1. Accreditation Council for Graduate Medical Education (ACGME) website, *www.acgme.org/outcome/comp/comp Full.asp.*
2. L. Edelstein, *The Hippocratic Oath* (Baltimore, Md.: Johns Hopkins Press, 1943).
3. Hippocrates, *On Surgery*, Harvard Classics (New York: P.F. Collier, 1910, 1915).
4. Aristotle, *Politics,* Book VII, Chapter XVI, for instance.
5. Both forms of the oath are found on a PBS website (WGBH/ NOVA): *www.pbs.org/wgbh/nova/doctors/oath_classical.html* and *www.pbs.org/wgbh/nova/doctors/oath_modern.html.*
6. A. Smith, *An Inquiry into the Nature and Causes of the Wealth of Nations* (London: Methuen & Co., 1789).
7. *http://content.healthaffairs.org.*
8. J. Fairbanks and W.H. Wiese, *The Public Health Primer* (Thousand Oaks, Calif.: Sage Publications, 1998), 23-5.
9. A problem of legitimacy might be noted: We were (through our representatives) given a chance to vote on the Clinton Plan; we don't remember voting to create the MCOs, which proceeded

directly from the FEMC.

10. "Medicare Choice," as it is called, was intended to bring the efficiencies of the free market to the provision of extended coverage (including pharmaceuticals) to the elderly. In Connecticut alone, almost 115,000 subscribed to Medicare Choice through one of seven HMOs, as of June 2000. *Connecticut Post,* 30 June 2000, C2.

11. At one point the insurance companies in Connecticut decided that there would be reimbursement for hospitalization after childbirth for only a 24-hour stay, which is fine for healthy experienced moms, but inadequate for new mothers or for recovery after a long (but not complicated) childbirth. So the howls went to Hartford, the legislature passed a law saying that every insurance plan must allow for a 48-hour stay, and that's what everyone now gets, even those who don't need it.

12. "AMA position paper on antitrust relief legislation," *www.ama-assn.org/ama/pub/category/12978.htm.*

13. G.C. Alexander et al., "Support for physician deception of insurance companies among a sample of Philadelphia residents," *Annals of Internal Medicine* 138, no. 6 (2003), cited in R.M. Werner, et al., "Lying to Insurance Companies: The Desire to Deceive among Physicians and the Public," *American Journal of Bioethics* 4, no. 4 (2004): 53-9.

14. M.K. Wynia et al., "Physician manipulation of reimbursement rules for patients: Between a rock and a hard place," *Journal of the American Medical Association* 283 (2000): 1858-65.

15. C. Feudtner, "Assuring Trust in Insurance," *American Journal of Bioethics* 4, no. 4 (2004): 64-6.

16. Especially L. M. Axtell-Thompson, "Back to Basics: Don't Lie, Cheat, or Steal," *American Journal of Bioethics* 4, no. 4 (2004): 66-9.

17. E.H. Morreim, "Gaming the System: Dodging the rules, ruling the dodgers," *Archives of Internal Medicine* 151, no. 3 (1991): 443-7; E.H. Morreim, *Balancing Act: The New Medical Ethics of Medicine's New Economics* (Washington, D.C.: Georgetown University Press, 1995).

18. Health Affairs website, *http://content. healthaffairs.org/content/vol0/issue2005.*

5

The Clinical Health Economics System Simulation (CHESS): A New Tool For Promoting Competency in Systems-Based Practice and Professionalism

John D. Voss, Natalie B. May, and Joel M. Schectman

In 1999 the American Council for Graduate Medical Education (ACGME) threw down the gauntlet for U.S. residency programs to move beyond teaching the usual medical knowledge and patient care skills to embrace competency-based education.[1] The move to competency-based education was not new, nor should it have been a surprise. Earlier calls for competency-based education were simply amplified by growing recognition[2] in the mid-1990s that teaching medical knowledge and patient care skills alone were insufficient preparation for the complex demands of practice.

In its mandate for competency-based education, the ACGME has identified six domains for physician competency. While the aforementioned medical knowledge and patient care skills are obvious subjects, the ACGME has increased the emphasis on professionalism and interpersonal and communication skills, and has added two new competencies — practice-based learning (PBL) and systems-based practice (SBP).[3] Residency programs across the country continue to wrestle with these new notions of competency, a challenge made greater because many medical educators possess only limited understanding of subjects like systems- and practice-based learning, let alone know how best to teach it. Even more vexing is the question of how to integrate teaching all the competencies, for the overlap between competencies, such as professionalism and systems-based practice, is wide and deep. While this could be perceived as an obstacle, this intersection of the competencies is useful, since it provides an opportunity for us to link and address some of the most important problems physicians and society must face. One central challenge is that we are developing technologies for improving health faster than their apparent incremental value in the midst of the demographic challenges of retiring baby boomers and rising numbers of uninsured patients.

Recognizing each specialty's need to develop unique solutions, the ACGME declined to specify the processes for arriving at the new state of competency-based education. Some clarity has emerged, however, among specialty organizations and training programs. Educators have begun to endorse the Dreyfus model of competency acquisition that has been promulgated by the ACGME,[4] which reflects the developmental nature of competence.[5] Residency programs have generated new learning objectives, or refined existing ones, to address these competencies,[6] and new teaching methods are appearing.[7] Competency assessment remains a major hurdle, but innovative solutions are in development.[8] Four of the six ACGME competencies pose special challenges. Medical knowledge and patient care skills are obvious subjects physicians-in-training must master; learners readily accept them, and educators have established curricula. The other four competencies require qualitatively different approaches. Systems-based practice is an exemplar of these challenges.

While the ACGME definition of systems-based practice includes many elements, competency in SBP fundamentally requires physicians to understand how the U.S. healthcare system is organized and financed, so that they can provide the highest value healthcare for patients and society. Embedded in this competency is a challenge to traditional concepts of medical professionalism, because the value one perceives in healthcare services varies as one's perspective shifts among patients, physicians, employers, insurers, and society. The trust patients place in physicians, however, is based on the assumption that physicians act to maximize patients' health without regard to the cost-effectiveness or incremental value of their efforts. When most everything a physician could do for a patient could be carried in a small black bag, this conflict between the individual, distributional equity and finite resources was mostly theoretical, or at least much less pronounced. As healthcare capabilities increase and costs spiral upward, this challenge has been recognized in documents such as the American Board of Internal Medicine charter on medical professionalism, that explicitly asks physicians to balance patient welfare and respect for patient autonomy with calls for an equitable distribution of scarce resources.[9] Unfortunately it is far easier to wax philosophic on paper than to teach physicians how to resolve this paradox in their daily practice.

These important subjects in medical education are far too often consigned to discussion at "liver rounds" after hours, rather than addressed in the formal medical curriculum. The challenges of educating learners about subjects such as systems-based practice and professionalism should not be underestimated. Resident physicians and medical students are bombarded daily with new information to assimilate; the task of learning patient care skills is cognitively and emotionally daunting; the pace of practice constrains physicians' attention to topics with immediate relevancy, and the culture of "Western" medicine eschews topics like SBP and professionalism.

From a pragmatic perspective, gaining competency in systems-based practice means acquiring knowledge and skills in practical health economics. Unfortunately, academic medical centers face numerous barriers training physicians in these new health management competencies.[10] Medical students, interns, and residents generally have little exposure to the realities of insurance and managed care,[11] nor of the impact of their clinical decisions on anything other than clinical outcomes. Most of the exposure that is provided in this area is generally in the form of an abstract lecture or didactic session. Since such presentations have little direct relation to the learners' current clinical needs and experience, they are generally poorly attended to, or soon forgotten. Instead of understanding the genesis of our current healthcare system, with its conflicting incentives, tensions, and trade-offs, learners are imbued with a visceral distrust of payers and administrators, stemming from the internal learning and role-modeling that occurs during training. At the same time, they are often exposed to a disease-enriched, predominantly hospitalized patient population, which reinforces their inclination to diagnostic and therapeutic intervention.[12]

WHY SIMULATION?

Within our own training program in Internal Medicine at the University of Virginia, we have addressed the requirements for competency-based education in disciplines like systems-based practice with several different methods. Our preferred method is to create novel participatory learning experiences that bring the relevance and value of these competencies into sharp focus. Given the difficulties that confound teaching competencies like SBP and professionalism, we felt that a healthcare simulation offered advantages over traditional teaching methods.[13] Simulations enable teachers to create events or structures that may not be available, or are only occasionally encountered by learners. Overly complex situations can be simplified to direct learners' attention to specific issues. Simulation variables can be employed to illustrate the influence of various parameters in healthcare decision making, such as out-of-pocket patient cost, or illness severity. Simulations, particularly when conducted in a team format, may provide a more engaging learning experience. In this chapter we will describe the simulation approach we have developed to teach the health economic aspects of systems-based practice to medical students and residents.

CHESS GOALS AND OBJECTIVES

We created the Clinical Health Economics System Simulation (CHESS) to allow resident physicians to view the effects of their clinical decision making on the less obvious nonclinical outcomes, since residents are exposed almost exclusively to purely clinical outcomes in most training programs. It is a computerized simulation of a healthcare delivery system that learners experience as teams working through clinical scenarios that provide them with the opportunity to discuss the subjects of practical health economics. The goals of CHESS are to teach residents and medical students to:

Clinical Health Economics System Simulation: A New Tool

1. Identify key components, relationships, and policies that comprise the structure, delivery, and financing of U.S. healthcare;
2. Understand how the decisions that healthcare professionals and patients make influence the costs of care for patients and society and the income of physicians;
3. Describe the concept of "value" in healthcare and the factors that lead physicians to provide care of greater or lesser value;
4. Identify, analyze, and resolve potential ethical conflicts created by the U.S. healthcare delivery and financing system.

CHESS is designed to accomplish teaching a variety of specific practical health economics objectives as enumerated in table 5.1.

Table 5.1
Clinical Health Economics System Simulation Objectives

To provide learners with the opportunity to:
1. Review common clinical scenarios where alternative decisions are clinically appropriate but have differing financial outcomes
2. Understand the different payer methods (fee-for-service vs. capitated payment models with variable provider financial risk) used in the U.S. healthcare system
3. Experience the impact of different payer mechanisms on medical decision making, clinical patient care, and costs for physicians, patients, and society
4. Review the effect of geography and extent of managed-care market penetration on reimbursement issues
5. Understand current prescription drug benefits and their impact on practices and costs
6. Assess the impact of patient case mix on decision making and outcomes for different payer mechanisms
7. Discuss tools and criteria that insurers utilize to evaluate/reimburse clinical decisions (level of care guidelines, prior authorization criteria, etc.)
8. Consider impact of clinical guidelines, patients' expectations, or preferences on medical decision making and costs
9. Engage in ethics discussions regarding coverage, decision making, economic perspective.

Adapted with permission from J.D. Voss, M.M. Nadkarni, and J.M. Schectman, "The Clinical Health Economics System Simulation," *Academic Medicine* 80, no. 2 (February 2005): 129-34, lists 1 and 2, and table 2. © 2005, Lippincott Williams & Wilkins, all rights reserved.

HOW CHESS WORKS

CHESS is designed as a small group activity for groups of three to 12 residents or medical students. Learners play the simulation grouped into three teams, each team representing a physician practice that is reimbursed under either one of two capitated methods or under a fee-for-service payment method.

Each team takes care of a panel of patients with a mixture of relatively healthy, moderately ill, or severely ill patients. The three teams of learners view each specific case and select one of two or three different treatments. These choices (more or less resource intensive) represent a style of patient care that the simulation uses to model the treatment intensity decisions that physicians would make for their panel over the year. For example, if faced with a congestive heart failure patient with an acute exacerbation who could reasonably be admitted or treated as an outpatient with medications and more frequent follow-up care, a team's decision to admit the patient is taken to represent a more resource intensive style of practice for other, similarly ill, patients.

The learners view each scenario together, and each team picks a treatment option for each case. The cases feature "toss-ups," such that all of the choices are medically justifiable yet have very different financial and utilization implications. CHESS gives learners immediate feedback on the patient and societal costs, as well as their own income, which will differ depending on the treatment selected and the team's method of reimbursement. This information is displayed in graphic and tabular form on the screen. If learners change treatments, the simulation displays immediate new feedback on all three costs.

The focus of each scenario differs to cover the learning objectives outlined in table 5.1. The faculty facilitator uses each case scenario to engage the learners in discussion about issues ranging from prescription formularies and patient co-payments to physician-induced demand. The simulation incorporates many of these topics as variables, allowing the learner to perform sensitivity analyses on their impact on income and costs. The ability to change variables like case-mix, panel size, and payment amounts and observe the effect on physician income, patient, and societal costs creates interest and learning ("If I'm paid FFS and you are paid capitation, how do our incentives to practice differ when a very ill patient walks in the door?") A partial list of variables is provided in table 5.2.

AN EXAMPLE SCENARIO

The GERD (gastroesophageal reflux disease) scenario is presented as an example in figure 5.1. Initially only the case and treatment options are visible. After the teams read the case, they discuss the available treatment options before announcing their selection. When each team's treatment choice is entered in the "Enter Treatment Selection" boxes, the graph and table shown in figure 5.1 register and can be selected for view. These elements display the primary care physician income for the year

Table 5.2
Simulation Variables

CHESS contains two variable types. Simulation level variables affect all scenarios and scenario level variables apply only within a specific scenario. Simulation level variables are further specified into subvariables that can vary by reimbursement type. Simulation variables include:
- Total panel size
- Case-mix (percent low, medium, or high severity patients)
- General overhead
- Malpractice overhead
- Total capitation per member (patient) per month (pmpm) rates for primary care services
- Percent of total monthly capitation at risk
- Geographic location (indirectly via differences in Medicare payment or capitation rate)
- Outpatient E&M Fee-For-Service Fee schedule adjustment as a percent of Medicare
- Physician work week (# weeks/ year, # sessions/week, # hours/session).

Scenario level variables include:
- Costs of tests such as upper endoscopy (GERD scenario)
- Costs of drugs utilized within each scenario (anti-hypertensives, proton pump inhibitors, inhalers, etc.)
- Baseline hospitalization costs (COPD scenario)

Adapted with permission from J.D. Voss, M.M. Nadkarni, and J.M. Schectman, "The Clinical Health Economics System Simulation," *Academic Medicine* 80, no. 2 (February 2005): 129-34, lists 1 and 2, and table 2. © 2005, Lippincott Williams & Wilkins, all rights reserved.

per patient, the estimated total (direct and indirect) costs per patient, and the estimated societal cost per patient for each of the three teams. A rich learner-centered, faculty-facilitated review of these outcomes follows using discussion questions as prompts, as needed. As learners discuss the case, they change treatment selections, patient co-payment amounts, drug costs, or other variables as desired for additional learning. The other scenarios (hypertension and chronic obstructive pulmonary disease — COPD) are similarly constructed.

After the three teams have reviewed all three cases they view the summary page (figure 5.2). The summary page displays graphs that extrapolate patient and societal costs and physician income for a one year, based on the payment method and treatment selections of each team. Learners have the opportunity to change overhead, malpractice costs, capitation rates, and fee-for-service (FFS) payment schedules, based on a percent of Medicare to see the effect of these changes on financial outcomes for patients, physicians, and society.

THE SCENARIO STRUCTURE

CHESS utilizes three common primary care scenarios (cases). We have selected clinical problems for scenario development based on the principle of "clinical equipoise," as defined as a medical condition with at least two medically justifiable treatment choices that can be expected to have substantially different financial implications for physicians, patients, or society. It is important to construct cases as medical "toss-ups," to minimize the amount of time medical learners spend debating the best medical choice, as well as to provide them with a case where they feel ethically justified to make a treatment decision on something other than the perceived best medical treatment.

To determine the financial outcomes of the treatment selected, each scenario is constructed with underlying decision trees that calculate the costs and health services that are consumed. The probabilities and outcome states that the decision trees utilize are drawn from the medical literature or come from the values for variables specified by simulation participants. Our initial simulation is constructed to run in Excel 97 or later versions, with a web-based simulation in development.

GERD: A LOW SEVERITY OF ILLNESS SCENARIO

It is your first day practicing as an attending physician. Your very first patient is a 38-year-old man with a 10-year history of moderate GERD. He does have daily symptoms that are of mild intensity and unchanged. He currently uses over-the-counter antacids 3 to 5 times per week. He has no alarm symptoms such as weight loss, sign/symptoms of gastrointestinal bleeding, use of NSAIDs. He specifically denies a history of peptic ulcer disease. The remainder of his history is unremarkable and his physical examination is normal.

Available treatment options:

1.	Advise him about non-pharmacologic measures to treat his GERD, prescribe a PPI, and suggest patient step down to PRN ranitidine in 4 to 8 weeks.
2.	Advise him about non-pharmacologic measures to treat his GERD, and give him a prescription for a proton pump inhibitor to take daily.
3.	Advise him about non-pharmacologic measures to treat his GERD, prescribe a proton pump inhibitor, and refer him for esophagogastroduodenoscopy.

Enter treatment selection:

Fee-for service	Capitation lower risk	Capitation higher risk
3	2	1

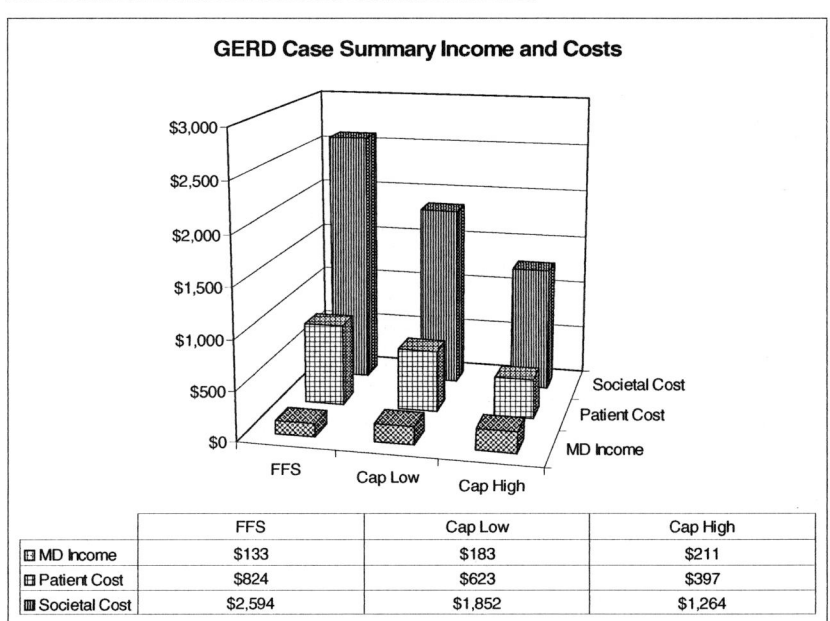

Figure 5.1.

MODELS OF COST

In each scenario three costs are modeled. First, the cost of primary care physician reimbursement is presented as physician income. The FFS team earns income based on how often

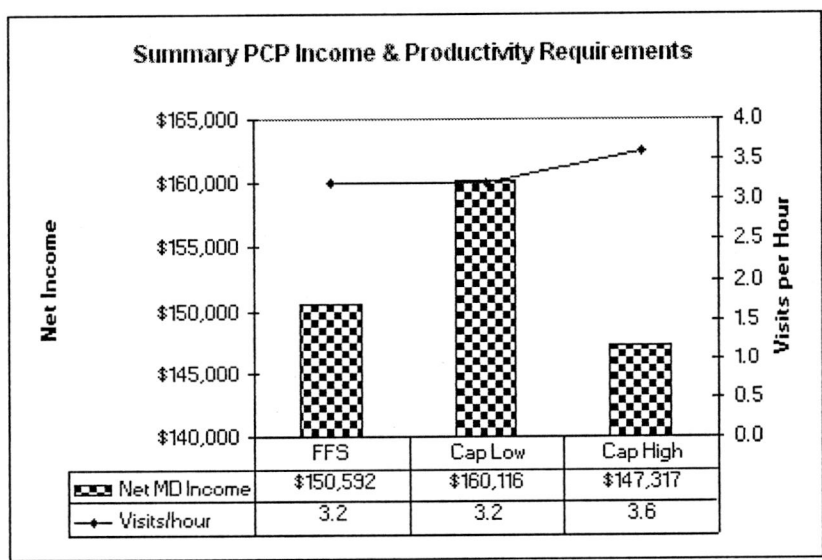

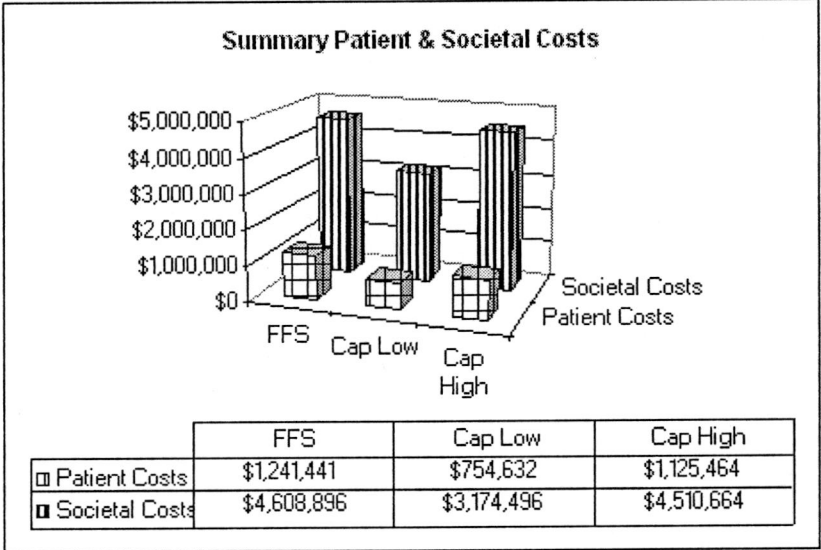

Figure 5.2.

and how intensively physicians treat patients. The simulation payment amounts for FFS physicians are a blend of current Medicare reimbursement for Evaluation and Management Services that can be further customized by simulation participants. Capitated physicians receive a per-member-per-month (pmpm) income based on panel size and a predetermined pmpm rate. Each capitated team also designates a fraction of their monthly capitation that is withheld to be paid based on the utilization decisions the teams make in each case. In the base case, one capitated team (cap low) assumes a very low risk (5 percent of pmpm is withheld) while the other team (cap high) assumes a higher degree (20 percent of pmpm) of risk. At the end of the simulation, each team has the opportunity to change their risk allocation to observe its effect on income and cost. Teams may not lose more than the withheld amount (a known/fixed downside risk), but may earn substantially more than the withheld amount. All physicians earn income from patient visit co-payments, and the simulation assumes a 100 percent collection rate for all physicians. All of these and multiple other variables can be adjusted to examine their effect on the summary cost outcomes for physicians, patients, and society.

To increase verisimilitude, the simulation counts how much physician work (in visits/per hour) each treatment choice, panel size, case-mix, or other selection creates. At the conclusion, CHESS shows participants how hard they have to work to generate the income and costs displayed. Learners who make poor choices (churning patient visits to increase income) get a slap in the face when the simulation estimates that they must see an distressingly high number of patients to generate their unrealistically high income.

PATIENT AND SOCIETAL COSTS

CHESS also simulates the patient cost of healthcare. This amount includes all direct out-of-pocket costs for office visits, prescriptions, and emergency and hospitalization co-payments, and also includes indirect costs, estimated as a variable fraction of direct costs. Indirect cost modeling serves as a method for introducing learners to the definition and significance of indirect costs. All patient costs are modeled as variables, and the aggregate patient costs are presented as outcomes.

The last costs modeled in each scenario are societal costs. These costs include elements from the two prior categories, but also include cost estimates for specialty care, hospitalization, home health, emergency room, and prescription costs over and above patient co-payment amounts, among others. While necessarily incomplete, these estimates of societal costs do provide an introduction to the societal perspective on costs, and why they are critical to consider in discussions of health policy. Because the simulation models costs over a one-year time period only, no future costs or discounting is modeled.

EARLY EXPERIENCE WITH CHESS

We have used CHESS to teach systems-based practice and professionalism in two primary settings. At a national meeting to promote education in systems-based practice and practice-based learning, we used CHESS with 72 internal medicine residents and faculty participating in the Achieving Competency Today grant program. These individuals represented 18 internal medicine programs across the United States. A post-test survey was conducted, with a 94 percent response rate regarding the simulation's utility as a learning instrument. Responses were highly favorable, as portrayed in table 5.3.

We have also conducted the CHESS simulation with 240 third-year medical students participating in a clinical skills development curriculum within an ambulatory internal medicine clerkship. We have conducted a preliminary analysis of 204 students based on pre- and post-simulation anonymous questionnaires examining participants' attitudes, beliefs, and self-reported knowledge about health economics. Survey questions were adapted from Simon and colleagues' survey of healthcare professionals' attitudes toward managed care, to ask each participant to rate whether capitated payment was superior; FFS was superior; they perceived no difference; or they did not know enough to express an opinion.[13] Questions included beliefs about which payment method would promote a better doctor-patient relationship, create more ethical conflicts, promote better quality of care, better continuity of care, improved chronic illness care, and offer the best care for a fixed amount of money. For each question a pre-post comparison using an exact test monte carlo method with 100,000 simulations was performed. Compared to their pretest responses, participants significantly changed their responses post-test in all cases, with p values ranging from 0.037 to < 0.0001. The greatest change in post-test assessments was for ethical conflicts, where 62 percent of respondents changed their assessment post-test, and the smallest de-

Table 5.3
CHESS Internal Medicine Resident and Faculty Evaluation

	Summary Mean	Standard Deviation
Managed-care kowledge and attitude ratings		
Self-rated managed-care knowledge (1=almost none, 5=very high)	2.9	0.13
Self-rated feelings towards managed care (1=very negative, 5=very positive)	2.7	0.10
Simulation learning objectives rating (1 = not helpful, 5 = very helpful)		
The effect of different payment mechanisms on physicians' income	4.45	0.078
The effect of payment mechanisms on the nature/cost of care patients receive	4.38	0.091
The effect of payment mechanisms on nature/cost of care society obtains	4.23	0.098
The potential effect on physician medical decision making	4.23	0.096
The impact of case mix and other variables on costs/income	4.32	0.088
The tools/methods used by MCOs to manage care (formularies, utilization review criteria)	4.00	0.101
The impact of physicians' decisions on healthcare costs	4.53	0.076
Simulation mechanics rating (1 = not useful, 5 = very useful)		
Use of clinical scenarios with "toss-up" decisions	4.50	0.064
Team-based approach to play	4.22	0.110
Quasi-competitive approach (e.g., play to "win")	3.30	0.155
Use of variables to perform sensitivity analyses on outcomes	4.36	0.084

Adapted with permission from J.D. Voss, M.M. Nadkarni, and J.M. Schectman, "The Clinical Health Economics System Simulation," *Academic Medicine* 80, no. 2 (February 2005): 129-34, lists 1 and 2, and table 2. © 2005, Lippincott Williams & Wilkins, all rights reserved.

gree of change was for value for the money, where only 48 percent of respondents changed their assessments. Pretest student "do not know" responses averaged approximately 30 percent, and can be assumed to represent a significant contribution to the change in attitudes and beliefs seen. Students rated their CHESS experience highly, with 88 percent reporting that they prefer the CHESS simulation to a lecture format presentation of this material, 7 percent prefer a combination of CHESS and lecture and 4 percent prefer a lecture, without the CHESS simulation.

CONCLUSION

Our experience with CHESS indicates that learners are eager to gain competence in the new or newly emphasized competencies like SBP and professionalism when they are presented in a relevant and engaging manner. The data thus far suggests that the use of cognitive simulations like CHESS are not only acceptable, but may be preferable to traditional teaching modalities. CHESS is a useful tool for promoting discussion at different levels of competence with no difference in the relatively high levels of satisfaction with CHESS-associated learning between attendings, residents, and students. Respondents have also indicated a willingness to use the simulation more than once if additional scenarios were available.

The generalizability of our conclusions is limited by the fact that our data is drawn from our experience as developers of the simulation conducting workshops with a product we know well. Because we developed the initial version of CHESS for our own use, it includes only modest educational support in the form of a 35-page teacher's guide and Powerpoint presentations. At present we are developing a web-based version with an improved set of learning objectives, educational support, and a competency assessment instrument. Upon completion, this version will be available free of charge to other institutions. An additional limitation is that our data does not indicate whether these changes in attitudes are sustained or give us insight into how physicians will negotiate the conflicts we have described. We are evaluating the potential of CHESS to answer these questions. We hope that instruments like CHESS and similar learning tools we are developing can promote the type of vigorous discussion and learning necessary to effect competency-based education.

ACKNOWLEDGMENTS

This work was supported by the University of Virginia Innovations in Graduate Medical Education program and the Partnership for Quality Education, a Robert Wood Johnson-sponsored initiative.

NOTES

1. P. Batalden et al., "General Competencies and Accreditation in Graduate Medical Education," *Health Affairs* 21, no. 5 (September-October 2002): 103-11.
2. M.J. Yedidia, C.C. Gillespie, and G.T. Moore, "Specific Clinical Competencies for Managing Care: Views of Residency Directors and Managed Care Medical Directors," *Journal of the American Medical Association* 284 (2000): 1093-8; N. Lurie, "Preparing Physicians for Practice in Managed Care Environments," *Academic Medicine* 71 (1996): 1044-9.
3. Accreditation Council for Graduate Medical Education, "ACGME Outcome Project: ACGME General Competencies Vers. 1.3 (9.28.99)," *http://www.acgme.org/outcome/comp/compFull. asp,* accessed 17 December 2003.
4. D.C. Leach, "Changing Education to Improve Patient Care," *Quality in Health Care* 10, suppl. 2 (2001): 54-8; G. Ogrinc et al., "A Framework for Teaching Medical Students and Residents about Practice-based Learning and Improvement, Synthesized from a Literature Review," *Academic Medicine* 78, no. 7 (2003): 748-56.
5. D.C. Leach, "Competence is a Habit," *Journal of the American Medical Association* 287, no. 2 (2002): 243-4.
6. D.M. Chapman et al., "Integrating the Accreditation Council for Graduate Medical Education Core Competencies into the Model of the Clinical Practice of Emergency Medicine," *Annals of Emergency Medicine* 43, no. 6 (June 2004): 756-69; P.L. Dyne, R.W. Strauss, and S. Rinnert, "Systems-based Practice: The Sixth Core Competency," *Academic Emergency Medicine* 9, no. 11 (November 2002): 1270-7; S.R. Hayden, S. Dufel, and R. Shih, "Definitions and Competencies for Practice-based Learning and Improvement," *Academic Emergency Medicine_*9, no. 11 (November 2002): 1242-8; B.D. Joyner, "An Historical Review of Graduate Medical Education and a Protocol of Accreditation

Council for Graduate Medical Education Compliance," *Journal of Urology* 172, no. 1 (July 2004): 34-9.

7. R.C. Ziegelstein and N.H. Fiebach, " 'The Mirror' and 'The Village': A New Method for Teaching Practice-based Learning and Improvement and Systems-based Practice," *Academic Medicine* 79, no. 1 (2004): 83-8; E. Allen et al., "Teaching Systems-based Practice to Residents by Using Independent Study Projects," *Academic Medicine* 80, no. 2 (2005): 125-8.

8. R.M. Epstein and E.M. Hundert, "Defining and Assessing Professional Competence," *Journal of the American Medical Association* 287, no. 2 (2002): 226-35; S.R. Swing, "Assessing the ACGME General Competencies: General Considerations and Assessment Methods," *Academic Emergency Medicine* 9, no. 11 (2002): 1278-88; C. Carraccio et al., "Shifting Paradigms: From Flexner to Competencies," *Academic Medicine* 77, no. 5 (2002): 361-7; C. Carraccio et al., "Educating the Pediatrician of the 21st Century: Defining and Implementing a Competency-based System," *Pediatrics* 113, no. 2 (February 2004): 252-8; A.G. Lee and K.D. Carter, "Managing the New Mandate in Resident Education: A Blueprint for Translating a National Mandate into Local Compliance," *Ophthalmology* 111, no. 10 (October 2004): 1807-12.

9. American Board of Internal Medicine, Project Professionalism, 1995, *http://www.abin.org/resources/publications/professionalism.pdf*, accessed 26 September 2005.

10. R. Kuttner, "Managed Care and Medical Education," *New England Journal of Medicine* 341 (1999): 1092-6.

11. A.V. Blue et al., "Incoming Primary Care Interns' Attitudes toward and Knowledge of Managed Care," *Academic Medicine* 74 (1999): S81-3.

12. K.M. Mazor et al., "Managed Care Education: What Medical Students Are Telling Us," *Academic Medicine* 77 (2002): 1128-33.

13. C.P. Friedman, "Anatomy of a Clinical Simulation," *Academic Medicine* 70 (1995): 205-9; J.L. Lane, S. Slavin, and A. Ziv, "Simulation in Medical Education: A Review," *Simulation & Gaming* 32 (2001): 297-314.

14. S.R. Simon et al., "Views of Managed Care — A Survey of Students, Residents, Faculty, and Deans at Medical Schools in the United States," *New England Journal of Medicine* 340 (1999): 928-36.

Internal Patient Care and Business Processes

6

Business Practices, Ethical Principles, and Professionalism

Ann E. Mills and Mary V. Rorty

INTRODUCTION

Whether in single practice, research organizations, government facilities, or complex hospitals or clinics, physicians practice in organizations. They are influenced by, and influence, the internal business practices of the organizations with which they are affiliated, as well as the business practices of other organizations that are part of the delivery system. It has always been true that the way in which care is delivered involves business practices. Healthcare delivery, whatever the model, is a business that involves costs and reimbursement issues. If there was earlier some hope that professional business practices did not require constant ethical re-examination because of the relative autonomy of the physician as professional, the radical restructuring of the healthcare system and the way healthcare has come to be reimbursed in the last two decades has brought into greater salience the impact of systemic business practices on professional practice.

The Accreditation Council for Graduate Medical Education (ACGME) acknowledges in its standards the interrelation of professionalism and business practices.[1] In the competencies on professionalism and systems-based practice listed in the ACGME Outcome Project,[2] ethical professional practice is placed in the context of the larger system within which the physician practices. If ethical professional standards are reflected in appropriate business practices, then the outcomes of the healthcare system as a whole may also be professionally responsible. But professional goals and the business practices designed to achieve them are not necessarily correlated throughout a healthcare system. Individual professionals may not have enough control, either of the institutions in which they practice or in the healthcare system as a whole, to assure ethically appropriate results. Furthermore, in any business practice, there are design characteristics that must be considered. If we want physicians to commit to standards that have been associated with professionalism, then the systems within which they work, and the business practices that are designed to achieve the goals of those systems, must support their activities as professionals. This can be achieved only if we design systems that are responsive to professional values and are characterized by some degree of flexibility. Business practices are not static, and the healthcare delivery system is fragmented. Each component, on each level — individual physicians, healthcare organizations, the payers and managed-care organizations that interact with them — has a plurality of values and goals that are supported by their own business practices. The more responsibility that is entrusted to professionals, the greater the temptation may be for other components of the delivery system to design intersecting practices that may corrupt or be perceived as corrupting professionalism.

In this essay, we look at the ACGME competencies on professionalism and systems-based practice, and consider the goals and values that they presuppose and the practices associated with them: the means by which organizations or individuals achieve their corporate or individual ends. We concentrate on business practices, defined broadly as relationships, processes, or procedures designed to meet some goal or produce some outcome. We demonstrate that each component of a business practice — its goal, the relationships or interactions which it encompasses, as well as the outcomes it produces — should be scrutinized for the ethical principles on which it relies as well as its effects on the other components. We focus our remarks at the organizational level of the delivery system, but they can apply to the micro level of the individual practitioner, and to the macro level of the objectives of the system as a whole. We address questions of what business practices are, how they are linked to goals and outcomes, and how they are designed in order to understand how threats to professionalism may arise through them. While business practices are a necessary condition for professional activity, they may be a source of problems as well. The problems faced by an ethical individual within an unethical system are not new or unique to medicine, but they do call attention to the impropriety of holding individuals responsible for systemic failings. We conclude that enlarging the concept of professionalism to include greater consideration of cost will not be enough for physicians and the organizations with which they are affiliated to achieve the goals of the competency on systems-based practice. For this, we may need to require that the system as a whole commit to the same goals.

THE ACGME COMPETENCIES

The competency on professionalism provided by the ACGME invites this re-examination. It states:

> Residents must demonstrate a commitment to carrying out professional responsibilities, adherence to ethical principles, and sensitivity to a diverse patient population. Residents are expected to:
>
> - demonstrate respect, compassion, and integrity; a responsiveness to the needs of patients and society that supersedes self-interest; accountability to patients, society, and the profession; and a commitment to excellence and ongoing professional development
> - demonstrate a commitment to ethical principles pertaining to provision or withholding of clinical care, confidentiality of patient information, informed consent, *and business practices* [authors' italics]
> - demonstrate sensitivity and responsiveness to patients' culture, age, gender, and disabilities[3]

The requirement of the ACGME that physicians "demonstrate a commitment to ethical principles pertaining to . . . *business practices*" as a condition for professionalism is a demand that physicians run their practices or operate their clinics or perform research in a way that is consonant with their professional ethics, and that they resist practices that prevent or distort their professional judgment. This competency calls for residents and other physicians to make a commitment to the ethical principles that pertain to medical ethics, clinical ethics, and "business practices." It is a three-pronged approach that acknowledges business practices are related to professionalism, and so may influence the way in which care is delivered.[4]

The ACGME competency on systems-based practice states:

Residents must demonstrate an awareness of and responsiveness to the larger context and system of health care and the ability to effectively call on system resources to provide care that is of optimal value. Residents are expected to:

- understand how their patient care and other professional practices affect other health care professionals, the health care organization, and the larger society and how these elements of the system affect their own practice
- know how types of medical practice and delivery systems differ from one another, including methods of controlling health care costs and allocating resources
- practice cost-effective health care and resource allocation that does not compromise quality of care
- advocate for quality patient care and assist patients in dealing with system complexities
- know how to partner with healthcare managers and health care providers to assess, coordinate, and improve health care and know how these activities can affect system performance

The systems-based practice competency complements the professionalism competency by emphasizing the integration and interconnections between different levels of the healthcare system and various sites of care. It recognizes that physicians practice at every level of the delivery system, and that physicians are constrained to act as the patient's advocate within that system. Differences in requirements, procedures, regulations, or business practices in the organizations with which practitioners interact affect their ability to exercise their professional judgment on behalf of their patients.

In the systems-based practice competency, the ACGME reiterates the overarching professional goal and desired outcome for physicians and whatever system within which they practice: to deliver care of optimal value. The professionalism competency requires that professionalism include a commitment to the ethical principles of business practices, and the systems-based practice competency supplies the goal toward which those business practices are coordinated.

WHAT ARE BUSINESS PRACTICES?

Business practices are the way in which people, resources, and technology are brought together to try and fulfill the values and goals of an organization. Interactions — relationships or procedures, processes or systems, policies or activities — can be examined as "business practices," depending upon the context in which they occur and the role they play in the operations of an organization or physician practice. Business practices may be formal or informal, simple or complex, but they exist only to fulfill the organization's goals. (An organization leader would be hard pressed to justify any business practice that does not in some way fulfill a goal associated with the organization.) They are designed and implemented to produce desirable organizational outcomes by affecting the behavior and decision making of internal or external stakeholders, either individuals or other organizations.

ETHICAL PRINCIPLES AND BUSINESS PRACTICES

Business practices are linked to organizational goals and have normative content. Most organizations produce either a product or a service for an identified customer or population of customers. Even government agencies can be so described, if the customer is seen as society as a whole. Many organizations want to keep their existing customers and add new customers, which they can only do if their products or services meet the standards expected by their customers. As a matter of course, they expect to be reimbursed for their efforts.

In the process of producing goods and services, maintaining and adding to their customer base, and collecting the revenue associated with the delivery of goods and services, organizations accrue costs, which, if not controlled, may threaten their viability. From this perspective, the business practices employed by any organization that wants to remain viable over the long term can be said to support three important organizational goals: product or service excellence, customers' satisfaction, and cost control. These goals are appropriate for healthcare organizations. Costs must be controlled, professional excellence must be maintained, and care must be delivered that is adequate or at least in some way satisfies the needs and expectations of patients and the community served by the healthcare organization. These goals are all associated either directly or indirectly with the long-term financial viability of the organization, as are the business practices that support them.

Each of these goals reflects ethical principles, insofar as they are associated with values that are endorsed by society. But the business practices associated with them may not reflect commonly accepted ethical principles, or may result in unethical outcomes. We believe it is unethical to produce goods under "sweat shop" conditions in order to control costs, but sweatshops do exist.[5] We do not believe it is ethical to allow known safety hazards in the production and supply of goods and services, but unsafe products have been known to be used or marketed.[6] Nor do we believe that unethical business practices should be used to achieve customers' satisfaction; for instance, clients are not allowed to dictate their wishes to auditors, regardless of the desirable effect on customers' satisfaction, when the practices they recommend are illegal or improper.[7] In the healthcare context, we question the conditions under which some professionals have been known to work,[8] we believe it is unethical for professionals to claim knowledge or skills they do not possess,[9] or for healthcare organizations to use unsafe practices, such as reusing needles.[10] Further, medical professionals are obligated not to harm their patients — whatever patients may wish.

Just as goals and business practices may not be correlated with ethical principles, practices and outcomes may not be correlated with ethical principles. This will depend on the design of the business practice in question and on the appropriateness of its use. For instance, a rigidly designed business practice that is employed in the manufacturing sector may be unethical if it employed in a professional setting. A tightly controlled quality initiative that employs detailed rules to govern every aspect of behavior and decision making may be inappropriate and reduce the quality of outcomes when it is implemented in an emergency room setting, which requires a great deal of individual discretion and professional judgment for success.

We have said that the goals of an organization may not reflect ethical principles when they are not associated with values endorsed by society. This very much depends on the form and function of the organization and society's expectations of it. For instance, although both for-profit and nonprofit healthcare organizations must remain viable, we have different expectations of the two types of organizations, and are disconcerted if we encounter behaviors accepted in the one in the other. We do not expect nonprofits to endorse the goals that are more commonly associated with for-profits, such as excessive profitability or market dominance.[11] The collapse of the Allegheny Health, Education, and Research Foundation (AHERF) is a case in point. Not only did it highlight the need for attention to roles and responsibilities of the various actors involved in the collapse, it raised questions about the appropriateness of those responsible for a community asset embarking on an aggressive strategy of horizontal and vertical integration.[12]

But ethically questionable goals that are endorsed by an organization may be associated with ethical business practices and ethical outcomes. A nonprofit healthcare organization that seeks market dominance may employ ethically appropriate business practices that deliver ethically appropriate outcomes. For instance, market pressures have forced many nonprofit religiously affiliated healthcare organizations to merge or consolidate with secular organizations to maintain their financial viability, or vice versa. Such combinations provide challenges for institutions that have been historically unwilling to provide services offered by their new partners. But while there has been controversy over the provision or discontinuation of specific services, centering on abortion and birth control, there is wide recognition that many mergers that involve Roman Catholic institutions have succeeded in improving the quality of care for the communities they serve.[13]

Equally, ethically questionable business practices and ethically questionable outcomes may be associated with ethically questionable goals. For instance, some question the ethical principles associated with the goal of Myriad Genetics, which is to obtain a worldwide monopoly on information pertaining to the BRCA1 breast cancer gene.[14] Just as questionable are Myriad's business practices and the outcomes associated with this goal. Myriad can command monopoly prices associated with tests for this breast cancer gene. This has resulted in the province of British Columbia discontinuing the use of the test because its healthcare system can not afford the $3,850 (Canadian dollars) price tag, which deprives women of a potentially important diagnosis option. So when we think about business practices, we have to think about the organizational goals they are designed to support, the way the business practices are designed and implemented, and the outcomes they produce and whether they are in alignment with community expectations. This leads to a matrix of possibilities in terms of the ethical principles associated with goals, business practices, and outcomes (see figure 6.1).

For physicians, the extent to which the goals, practices, or outcomes of the organizations with which they are affiliated support or contradict their professional values is crucial. Any of the three may constitute a possible threat to practitioners' professionalism and must be scrutinized by physicians regarding their influence on physicians' decision making. Physicians understand the need to maintain the financial solvency of their practices, or of the hospitals to which they admit. But physicians who prioritize excellence of practice may hesitate to associate their personal reputations with a healthcare organization that blatantly ignores the quality of care it provides in favor of high profits or one that consistently ignores patients' dissatisfaction.

ADDITIONAL COMPLICATIONS

There are further complications in trying to disentangle the ethical principles that are associated with organizational goals, the business practices that are meant to support them, and the outcomes they produce. Organizations, like individuals, typically have a pluralism of values and goals. Further, some practices that are appropriate to an agent at one level of a healthcare system may be perceived as inappropriate if exercised by other agents.

Most organizations or individual practices are committed to more than one goal. But these goals can conflict. Business practices that are designed to maximize potentially competing objectives require ongoing balance and prioritization to achieve their objectives. For instance, most organizations, including healthcare organizations, endorse both quality (meeting customers' expectations through product or service excellence to maximize customers' satisfaction) and cost-constraint as goals to be achieved. The potential for conflict between quality and cost is well known. Improved quality is often, although not always, associated with increased costs. Similarly, lower costs are often, although not always, associated with decreased quality. Many organizations assign priorities to the achievement of their goals. For instance, many organizations will place customer service or product excellence before cost, in the belief that profits depend more on these factors than on cost-control.[15] (Many organizations, including healthcare organizations, codify their priorities and the values they represent in mission statements, ethical codes, or value statements.) But it very well may be the case that two ethically acceptable goals, when reprioritized, produce ethically unacceptable business practices or outcomes. Or, it may be that the goals themselves, when reprioritized, are perceived as unethical, depending upon the wider social expectations of the business in question. For instance, we do not expect healthcare organizations to prioritize cost-control over adequate care, and when they do, we perceive it as unethical.

An additional complication is associated with the source of a business practice that might cause it, or its goals and outcomes, to be perceived as ethical or unethical. For instance, utilization review that is instigated by third-party insurers and used to con-

MATRIX OF POSSIBILITIES

Ethically acceptable = A   Ethically unacceptable = U

Goals	Practice	Outcomes
A	A	A
A	A	U
A	U	A
A	U	U
U	A	A
U	A	U
U	U	A
U	U	U

Figure 6.1.

trol physicians' decision making is widely perceived as unethical.[16] But if the utilization review is instituted by a hospital with its residents and physicians, it may be viewed as a nuisance or irritant, but may not be perceived as unethical by physicians. If it is done by peers, physicians might perceive it as an attempt to educate them concerning new evidence about specific diagnosis and treatment options. This is the case, even when utilization review purports to support the quality and cost goals of organizations. So, the exact same mechanism, used for exactly the same purpose, may be perceived as ethical or not depending on its source.

Business practices may also be subtle, with outcomes that are not tightly linked in time to the practice or the organizational goal they support. For instance, one well-known practice is the intrusion of drug company representatives who may attempt to endear themselves to residents or other physicians with invitations, goods, or services of various sorts.[17] A midnight pizza party may be harmless, but its intended outcome may not be so harmless, if the object is to capture the attention (and the gratitude) of the recipient, to be reciprocated by prescribing from the representative's company. So what may be perceived as a harmless business practice may not be so harmless, but rather subtle and invidious.

DESIGNING BUSINESS PRACTICES

Business practices, even when they are aligned with organizational goals that reflect generally accepted ethical principles, may be themselves unethical or may produce unethical outcomes. This will depend on how the practice is designed and whether or not its design is appropriate for the context in which it is implemented. Some tasks demand a great deal of precision, with little scope for variation. Others can be specified best in terms of their goals and some behavioral parameters, leaving the processes for their accomplishment up to the particular agent. An organization of any size that is designed to deliver healthcare must coordinate the actions and services of a number of different skilled and less-skilled workers, so the business practices that are associated with various organizational tasks must be appropriate to the demands of those tasks. So there is an important characteristic when considering the design of business practices: the amount of rigidity or flexibility they possess.[18]

An important distinction in the design of any business practice is whether or not it is largely mechanical (rigid) or naturally flexible. This distinction is fundamental and describes how a business practice is designed and how it responds to external or internal stimuli. In mechanical systems, we can predict in great detail the interaction of each of the parts in response to a given stimulus, since, in a purely mechanical system, pre-specified responses are always correct and a correct response is always expected. For instance, an organization might use mechanical assembly lines as part of its business practices. If all parts are working correctly, when it is turned on, the line begins to function as it was designed. When deviation occurs (for example, the line does not turn on) it is unexpected and generally provokes study (is a fuse blown?) and action to prevent recurrence (replacing the fuse). Another example is a tightly controlled quality control technique that requires exact measurements or very specific interactions among its components. These components may or may not be human beings.

It might well be the case that tightly controlled business practices do not have to be closely monitored for the production of potentially unethical outcomes. If the practice is ethically designed and it produces ethical outcomes, then it will, barring unforeseen events, always produce ethical outcomes. For instance, a tightly controlled and ethical billing process will always produce the same outcomes, and if it is designed to produce ethical outcomes, it will always produce ethically acceptable outcomes. But the context in which it is used may vary, and it is not always appropriate to use tightly controlled practices.

Other business practices must have more flexibility in their design. For instance, most healthcare organizations employ teams of personnel to evaluate, treat, and monitor individual patients. These teams are composed of administrators, case managers, doctors, nurses, social workers, chaplains, and others who work within the business practice of "case management" to produce one or more goal. Persons who are associated with the team must have some flexibility in how to best achieve the goals of case management, because each patient and her or his circumstances are unique, and it would be inappropriate (and probably disastrous) to try and rigidly govern the interactions of the team. Thus, we can think of business practices as falling somewhere on a continuum between the poles of extreme rigidity and extreme flexibility. This characteristic is important, not only because it is central to the design of a business practice, but also because the degree of flexibility of a business practice may determine the propriety of the business practice itself and its outcomes. For instance, when physicians set up practice, they must allow enough flexibility in time and other resources to accommodate patients with varying needs. When a hospital requires the use of evidence-based medicine in clinical decision making, rigid adherence to guidelines may itself be unethical, and may also produce unethical outcomes, depending on the values and preferences of the individual patient.[19]

Flexible business practices are needed when human judgment is required. But it should be noted that the flexibility of a business practice may allow its components, including human beings, through their interactions, to change either the practice itself or the goals it is intended to achieve.[20] Because either the goals or the practice can change through the interactions of its components, the ethicality of the practice or its outcomes cannot be guaranteed.

The characteristic of rigidity or flexibility will also determine whether or not additional business practices, such as incentives, are perceived to be needed to influence decision making. In our earlier example, if all parts of an assembly line are working correctly, as they are expected to do, desirable organizational outcomes will be produced. There is little need to provide additional incentives to produce these outcomes. But if an application requires more flexibility in the design of a business practice — if it requires the exercise of judgment, of skill, of intuition, of the interactions of varying individuals or groups — positive or negative incentives might be needed to align decision making with desirable organization outcomes. And, of course, incentives themselves can be flexible or not, depending on how closely linked they are to expected outcomes and how rigorously they are enforced.

PROFESSIONALISM

Professionals are expected to exercise their judgment on behalf of individuals or organizations. Their judgment, based on rigorous, esoteric study, and experience,[21] is expected to benefit the individual or organization with which the professional is associated, and also society as a whole. Engineers are expected to prioritize safety in the design of new products so that we, as members of society, can purchase and use these new products without undue fear. Physicians, lawyers, and priests are expected to have relationships with their patients, clients, and penitents that are based on trust, so that we, as a society, can believe that the sick, the legally challenged, and the sinner can find a safe haven where the individual's interests are ascertained, respected, and advocated for, through the judgment and the activities of the professional.

To practice the profession for which they have been trained, physicians will constitute themselves as, or associate themselves with, an organization that is in the business of delivering healthcare. Such an organization can be a sole practice, a partnership, or a clinic of several physicians; a healthcare organization; a research organization; a multi-practice clinic; or other entity, including government service or research institutions.[22] That organization will have goals, practices, and outcomes. Organizations that are constituted to facilitate the practice of medicine are not identical with the person of the practitioner. Practitioners are bound by the codes of the profession, but the organizations that physicians constitute or join as the context and the medium of their practice are the means through which physicians exercise their professional expertise in the service of patients. Organizations are "medical providers" or professional agents, but they are so in a secondary or derivative way, by association with professionals.

Healthcare organizations do not have a "professional ethic," but, since they are organizations of and for professional practice, they should be structured in a way that facilitates rather than impedes professional practice. Thus, practitioners must be conscious of, and scrutinize, the extent to which their sites of practice, healthcare organizations, will be appropriate means for the exercise of their profession — an efficient and effective means — one that facilitates the exercise of their professional obligations without presenting obstacles to ethical practice.

WHY AND HOW DO THREATS TO INDIVIDUAL PROFESSIONALISM EMERGE?

In this context, threats to the professional judgment of an individual emerge because the outcomes that are associated with professional judgment are deemed undesirable from the perspective of some individual or organization who is affected by it.

Either they are undesirable in themselves or they may conflict with other desirable outcomes or organizational goals. Threats can emerge from both the internal and external environment, and they can take the form of either a business practice or an incentive (which, as we have said, is another form of a business practice). Either or both can be associated with either the external or internal environment.

The larger society has been conflicted about the rising costs of healthcare in the United States, while it has been generally satisfied with the level of care available. In the late 1990s, a period now being called the "era of managed care," various business practices that were associated with reimbursement were introduced by payer organizations, on the assumption that the costs of care could be controlled without reducing the quality of care. Various restrictions and incentives were introduced in hopes of altering physicians' behavior. Some produced undesirable results because they attempted to externally constrain physicians' judgment.[23]

But professional judgment is perhaps the most important service offered by healthcare organizations. Because professional judgment depends on a number of different factors, some of which may be outside the organization's control, supporting it requires flexible business practices. If business practices are inappropriately rigid, such that professionals' judgment is constrained, inhibited, or influenced, these business practices can be seen as a threat to professionalism. In the above example, a tightly controlled quality technique, when applied in an emergency room setting, might be a threat to professionalism if rules are substituted when professional judgment is required. Other threats to professionalism can emerge through the use of incentives.

All incentives appeal to individuals' self-interest, and many incentives are quite straightforward. Individuals are rewarded by enhancing their performance within prescribed parameters. Enhancing individuals' performance is linked with enhancing an organization's performance. So there is a direct relationship between individuals' goals and the organization's goals. But because of some anomalies of healthcare (particularly the fact that the consumer of healthcare goods and services is not generally the payer),[24] excellent professional judgment may produce undesirable organizational outcomes: costs that are associated with preserving professional judgment may be perceived as excessive. Moreover, because healthcare systems include these kinds of anomalies, more than one stakeholder generally has a stake in the outcomes of professional judgment. Therefore, incentives in healthcare that are designed to affect professional judgment are more complex than they might be otherwise. Supporting professional judgment might mean increasing the likelihood of additional organizational costs. Thus, incentives may be designed that pose a conflict of interest or commitment for the professional — who is perceived to be the gateway to the costs incurred by the healthcare system and its components, and also the gateway to the profits to be made.

A *conflict of interest* refers to situations in which one's professional judgment or professional code is in conflict with other demands or influences that, if acted upon, would compromise professional judgment. An organizational demand that questions one's professional judgment or conflicts with a professional code creates the potential for one such type of conflict.

Conflicts of interest occur in every part of life, as various roles conflict with other roles, when professional integrity is at question, when there are professional biases concerning judgment, or when demands for financial rewards, cost-cutting, or greater efficiency challenge one's professional decision making. Having a conflict of interest itself, however, is not necessarily unethical. It is only when one acts on a conflict in ways that break acceptable rules for sound professional decisions, that jeopardize professional judgment, or that cause harm, that the conflict raises ethical issues.

Conflicts of interest are usually distinguished from conflicts of commitment, although they often overlap. According to Patricia Werhane and Jeffrey Doering, "Conflicts of commitment are those sets of role expectations where competing obligations prevent honoring both commitments or honoring them both adequately."[25]

All physicians face the possibility that the demands of care of one patient will threaten the care of the other patients for whom they are responsible. The profession of medicine itself incorporates care of the patient and advancement of medical science as possibly competing commitments. As professionals who have limited time and resources and a variety of professional demands, physicians are often faced with conflicting demands of their profession that are impossible to honor simultaneously. Conflicts of commitment also arise as role conflicts. In a complex society, each of us has a number of roles, and inevitably they clash. One simply cannot honor all one's commitments as a parent, spouse, citizen, professional, manager, and employee satisfactorily, all of the time. Unlike conflicts of interest, one can neither avoid the existence of conflicts of commitment nor avoid acting on those conflicts unless one simply abrogates all one's duties altogether. In all cases, however, the ability of professionals to ignore the conflict and base decisions purely on professional judgment depends on the amount of flexibility and the strength of incentives built into these practices. But if outcomes are not expected to be affected by the conflicts raised — and if enough flexibility allows professionals to ignore them and if incentives are diluted so that they are ineffective — why go to the time and trouble of creating them?

Organizations too face conflicts of interest and conflicts of commitment. One of the criticisms most frequently made of for-profit managed care is that the obligation to serve the patient, which constitutes and defines the social institution of healthcare, is in possible conflict with the need to make profits for shareholders. As the conversion of previously philanthropic foundations to for-profit healthcare institutions in the U.S. accelerates, the discussion grows more heated. What is not questioned is the requirement of fiscal responsibility: any healthcare institution must remain economically viable to fulfill its mission of delivering healthcare to the individuals and population for which it undertakes responsibility. The strategies, systems, or processes it uses to maintain that viability — in changing circumstances — present a shifting array of moral questions to committed practitioners.

EVALUATING BUSINESS PRACTICES, GOALS, AND OUTCOMES

Before individual physicians can commit to the ethical principles that pertain to business practices, they should evaluate the suitability of those principles for their practices, from the perspective of the goals of their organization, the priority of these goals, the design of their practice, and whether or not the design of the practice produces ethically acceptable outcomes. Therefore, physicians must have standards that can be used for purposes of evaluation. For this, physicians have traditionally looked to the standards that are associated with professionalism.

The traditional professional ethics of medicine has defined the duties of its practitioners in relation to activities that advance the best interest of the individual patient, within the context of a relationship based on mutual respect and trust. If we assume that the best interest of patients lies in the ability of physicians to exercise their professional judgment to deliver adequate care to patients, then business practices that prevent the exercise of professional judgment or inhibit it can be perceived as a threat to the professionalism of physicians — which we cannot ask physicians to support. But if the goal of physicians is to deliver care that is cost-effective, then we have added a new dimension to the concept of professionalism and to the professional obligations of physicians and hence to the evaluation of a business practice, its goals, and outcomes. It may be that when the provision of cost-effective care conflicts with the traditional obligations of physicians, some decisions should be made on the basis of cost-effectiveness.

Quality care (or at least adequate care) and cost-effectiveness are goals endorsed by society as ethically appropriate — with one caveat. Society deems the quality of care, which must include some aspects of professionalism, as more important than the cost of care. It views a reprioritization of these goals as ethically unacceptable.

But we know from our discussion of business practices that goals, the business practices that support them, and the outcomes they produce, may not reflect ethically desirable characteristics. We know from our discussion of the design of business practices that accommodating professionalism will require some degree of flexibility, and we know that flexibility cannot guarantee the achievement of specific goals. We also know that flexibility may invite interactions (business practices) from other components of the system that may not share the same goals, or may prioritize them differently. How do we prevent these goals from becoming reprioritized or distorted? How do we align business practices with outcomes so they reflect ethically desirable characteristics? Will expanding the obligations of physicians to consider cost-effective care be enough to ensure that they are able to deliver quality care at optimal value?

A SYSTEMS ETHIC?

The ACGME's professionalism competency emphasizes the individual physician's responsibility for professional practice, and the systems-based practice competency contextualizes this responsibility to the various organizations and practice options that constitute the larger healthcare system. Since most, if not all, medical practice occurs within some organizational context, individuals must be alert to possible conflicts of interest and commitment that can arise because of the plurality of goals that any organization must have in order to survive. But, because of the fragmentation of the healthcare system as currently constituted, it is possible that individual responsibility alone will be inadequate to prevent or avoid professionally undesirable outcomes.

Elsewhere we have advocated the formation of an organizational ethics program that, at least at the mid level of the system — the organizational level — might be helpful as a mechanism of intervention when a practitioner perceives the threat of inappropriate reprioritization or distortion of the goal of care of optimal value.[26] We have suggested that it is important that any healthcare organization's business practices should be aligned with its essential values and goals, and that that conflict be resolved by appeal to those goals and values. The healthcare organization exists to provide care, and, since care of high quality must reflect some degree of professionalism, there is no necessary or intrinsic conflict between the professional responsibilities of the individual physician and the organizations within which he or she practices. However, we also know that the business practices of the various components of the system interact together in ways that might reprioritize or distort these goals. If we want to achieve the goal of quality care of optimal value, if we want business practices to support professionalism, and if we want to achieve appropriate outcomes, then we must start at the systems level. This will require that the system, as a whole, commits to the same goal, as well as to principles that govern the way in which business practices interact and the outcomes they produce. Even then, this might not be enough to ensure the system achieves the results we want.

Supporting professionalism requires flexibility in business practices. The system as a whole must have the ability to react to unforeseen events, to negotiate when appropriate, and to problem-solve in a creative way. But flexibility in business practices, although a precondition for professionalism, cannot guarantee appropriate outcomes, nor can it guarantee that the practices themselves will not change. Therefore, even if the delivery system and all of its components commit to the same goal and to the same principles, its outcomes and its practices must be continuously reevaluated.

A persuasive argument could be made that implementing a code that governs the goals, interactions, and outcomes of a system, and a mechanism that monitors its implementation in delivery of healthcare services, is desirable both because it opens the door to increased efficiency and effectiveness and because it is the right thing to do. However, this is unlikely in the short-term. In the short-term the healthcare system will remain fragmented and open to abuses.

CONCLUSION

The professionalism and systems-based practice competencies of the ACGME Outcome Project combine to enlarge the professional obligations of residents (and by extension, all physicians) to greater consideration of costs in the delivery of care. That obligation may be enough to deliver some kind of care of optimal value, but it does not guarantee the preservation of professionalism as it has been traditionally understood. It may put residents in an untenable position relative to their patients. It may also further undermine the trust and respect that we as a society have for our physicians.

Quality in healthcare requires the provision of professional care, and this requires the ability of a system's professionals to exercise their judgment. Compromising that judgment through badly designed business practices or inappropriate financial incentives will not produce the results we want, if it undermines the patient-centered ethos that is central to good medical practice. The challenge to professionals, to the organizations with which they are associated, and to industry leaders is to design business practices that are capable of achieving cost-control goals while still standing the test of being evaluated against professional standards. This will require an integrated perspective that recognizes the legitimacy of organizational cost-control goals while it simultaneously gives priority to the quality goals of the practice or the healthcare organization.

The development of an integrated ethics for the healthcare system as a whole is a daunting task. In the short-term we can ask professionals to be aware of and to scrutinize an institution's goals, business practices, and outcomes for their effect on professionalism. We can endeavor to teach residents the importance of personal and professional integrity and can call their attention to the intricacies of the wider delivery system. We can urge attention to organizational ethics for help in resolving issues that healthcare organizations can control. These are the first steps toward the development of a successful delivery system. This, however, will not be enough for the future, unless the system as a whole is explicitly committed to these same principles. The alignment of values of individual and organizational agents, at all levels of a system, is the task to which leaders in medicine are committed. The ACGME competency standards on professionalism that require individual physicians to commit to the principles of medical ethics while they simultaneously commit to the ethical principles of business practices, represents a step toward developing such an integrated perspective among physicians.

ACKNOWLEDGMENT

The authors are indebted to Patricia Werhane for constructive review of this essay and to the Batten Institute of the Darden Graduate School of Business Administration at the University of Virginia for their support of our collaboration.

An earlier version of this chapter appeared in *Organizational Ethics: Healthcare, Business, and Policy*, volume 2, no.1 (Spring 2005). ©2005, University Publishing Group. Used with permission. All rights reserved.

NOTES

1. The ACGME is responsible for the accreditation of post-MD medical training within the United States. Accreditation is accomplished through a peer-review process and is based upon established standards and guidelines.

2. See *http://www.acgme.org/Outcome/* and retrieve the competencies under "Outcome Project," or see the appendix to this volume.

3. Most business practices can be investigated as systems. A "system" has been defined as "a complex of interacting components together with the relationships among them that permit the identification of a boundary-maintaining entity or process." See A. Laszlo and S. Krippner, "Systems Theories: Their Origins, Foundations and Development," in *Systems Theories and*

a Priori Aspects of Perception, ed. J. Scott (Amsterdam, the Netherlands: Elsevier, 1988), 51.

Systems are connected in ways that enhance the fulfillment of one or more goals or purposes. Systems may be micro (small, self-contained, with few interconnections) or macro (large, complex, consisting of a large number of interconnections and purposes). A system may be rigid and function mechanically, or it may be what Paul Plsek calls an "adaptive system," because it consists of individuals and organizations that have the liberty to interact with, respond to, and change the system. See P. Plsek, "Redesigning Health Care with Insights from the Science of Complex Adaptive Systems," in *Crossing the Quality Chasm: A New Health System for the 21st Century* (Washington D.C.: National Academy Press, 2001), 310-33.

4. This integration of clinical, professional, and business ethics is the definition of organizational ethics in E.M. Spencer et al., Organization Ethics in Healthcare (New York: Oxford University Press, 2000), chap. 12, pp. 200-10.

5. See *http://www.corpwatch.org/article.php?list=type &type=108* for a definition of sweatshops and a list of articles detailing recent cases.

6. See *http://cc.msnscache.com/cache.aspx?q=81476974579 &lang=en-US&FORM=CVRE7* for the infamous Ford Pinto memo in which costs to repair the back end of the Pinto were compared against anticipated deaths. See also G.T. Schwartz, "The Myth of the Ford Pinto Case," *Rutgers Law Review* 43 (1991): 1013.

7. Arthur Andersen's role in the collapse of Enron is especially notorious. For example see J.D. Glater, "Last Task at Andersen: Turning Out the Lights," *New York Times,* 30 August 2002 .

8. H.S. Berliner and E. Ginzberg, "Why This Hospital Nursing Shortage Is Different," *Journal of the American Medical Association* 288 (2002): 2742-4. See also S. Veasey et al., "Sleep Loss and Fatigue in Residency Training: A Reappraisal," *Journal of the American Medical Association* 288 (2002): 1116-24.

9. S. Rosenbaum, "The Impact of United States Law on Medicine as a Profession," *Journal of the American Medical Association* 289 (2003): 1546-56.

10. R. Voelker, "Eradication Efforts Need Needle-Free Delivery," *Journal of the American Medical Association* 281 (1999): 1879-81.

11. L.E. Singer, "The Conversion Conundrum: The State and

Federal Response to Hospitals' Changes in Charitable Status," *American Journal of Law and Medicine* 23 (1997): 221.

12. L.R. Burns et al., "Business of Health Care; The Fall of the House of AHERF: The Allegheny Bankruptcy; A chronicle of the hows and whys of the nation's largest nonprofit health care failure," *Health Affairs* (January-February, 2000).

13. J.M. Kellhofer, "American Pluralistic System: Mergers between Catholic and Non-Catholic Healthcare Systems," *Journal of Law and Health* 16, no. 103 (2001/2002), available at LexisNexis.

14. L.B. Andrews, Biotechnology Symposium: The Gene Patent Dilemma: Balancing Commercial Incentives with Health Needs," *Houston Journal of Health Law & Policy* 65 (2002). See also J. Paradise, "European Opposition to Exclusive Control Over Predictive Breast Cancer Testing and the Inherent Implication for U.S. Patent Law and Public Policy: A Case Study of the Myriad Genetics' BRCA Patent Controversy," *Food and Drug Law Journal* 59 133 (2004): 133. See also S. Gad et al., "Identification of a Large Rearrangement of the BRCA1 Gene Using Colour Bar Code on Combined DNA in an American Breast/Ovarian Cancer Family Previously Studied by Direct Sequencing," *Journal of Medicine and Genetics* (2001): 3888.

15. The idea that quality in the production of goods and services is paramount is the basis for the whole "quality" movement. The central idea is that if producers consistently examined their processes then costs would fall as quality rose. See W.E. Deming, "Improvement of Quality and Productivity Through Action by Management," *National Productivity Review* 1, no. 1 (Winter 1981-1982): 12-22. Also see R.W. Grant, R. Shani, and R. Krishnan, "TQM's Challenge to Management Theory and Practice," Sloan Management Review 35, no. 2 (1994): 25-35.

16. M.K. Wynia et al., "Physician Manipulation of Reimbursement Rules for Patients: Between a Rock and a Hard Place," *Journal of the American Medical Association* 238 (April 2000): 1858-65.

17. See Jerome P. Kassirer, *On the Take: How Medicine's Complicity with Big Business Can Endanger your Health* (New York: Oxford University Press, 2005), for a description of this and many other business practices that are designed to influence physicians' judgment.

18. Plesk, see note 3 above, pp. 310-33.

19. A.E. Mills and E.M. Spencer, "Evidence Based Medicine: Why Clinical Ethicists Should be Concerned," *HEC Forum* 15, no. 3 (Fall 2003): 231-44.

20. Plesk, see note 3 above.

21. Spencer et al., see note 4 above; see chapter 5 for a discussion of professionalism, pp. 69-91.

22. J.C. Robinson, *The Corporate Practice of Medicine* (Berkeley, Calif.: University of California Press, 1999).

23. J.C. Robinson, "The End of Managed Care," *Journal of the American Medical Association* 285 (2001): 2622-8.

24. This anomaly of the healthcare system was noted in 1995 by E. Haavi Morreim, who writes, "in this sense the term purchaser is systematically ambiguous; we could be referring either to patients or to payers." See E.H. Morreim, *Balancing Act: The New Medical Ethics of Medicine's New Economics* (Washington D.C.: Georgetown Press, 1995), 22.

25. P. Werhane and J. Doering, "Conflicts of Interest and Conflicts of Commitment," *Professional Ethics* 4 (1005): 47-82.

26. Spencer et al., see note 4 above, pp. 73-6.

7

Individuals, Systems, and Professional Behavior

Evan G. DeRenzo

INTRODUCTION

The Outcome Project of the Accreditation Council for Graduate Medical Education (ACGME) has set a difficult and important goal for residency programs.[1] Of its six general competencies, the inclusion of an explicit focus on systems-based practice is recognition of the radical changes needed to achieve excellence in medicine. Although the consideration of systems-based organizations has been gaining credibility for many years across a variety of fields, it has yet to be embraced in medicine.

Systems thinking represents a profound shift in understanding organizations and processes. Systems thinking rejects a mechanistic, reductionist understanding of organizations and processes in which the whole is thought to be merely the sum of the parts, in which the primary focus is on the nature of the part rather than the interactions between and across parts. Rather, systems thinking understands organizations and processes as interactive, with the parts as subsystems and the system itself as a part of a larger suprasystem. Systems thinking understands that the parts are not merely additive, but that they affect each other.

The whole is now understood to be far more than the sum of the parts.² Today, systems theories dominate the field of organizational science. One can even see systems thinking creeping into medicine. Healthcare organizations, such as Intermountain Health Care, apply systems-based practices to their healthcare delivery processes, resulting in excellence in patient outcomes.³ Juxtaposing systems thinking with traditional medical practice, however, is difficult for many. This may be because applying a systems approach can seem almost heretical to medicine's moral traditions.

At its heart, medicine is about the relationship of an individual physician to an individual patient. To be a physician, or at least a good one, is to take on the persona of healer, caregiver to the sick and the needy. To be a patient is to suffer, to feel pain and fear, to experience loss, to face death. To be a patient is to give up equality and to be forced to trust. These complex human experiences make the patient dependent on the skill, competence, compassion, and professionalism of his or her physician.

A contemporary perspective on the traditional doctor-patient relationship, however, encourages thinking of patients as customers or consumers, individuals entering into a contractual relationship for medical services. Thinking of patients this way is appealing. It is far less complex to construct morally acceptable roles in a relationship of equals than in one in which the weak is dependent on the stronger. But patients, especially the sick, frail, or frightened, will never be equal partners entering into an exchange of goods and services such as one does when buying a loaf of bread or a new car. The conditions of need that bring a patient to a doctor are inequality in health, knowledge, and power.

Appreciation of the dangers for abuse from the unequal power distribution of this relationship has produced centuries of scholarship and professional attention to building protections for patients into the doctor-patient relationship. Now, into the ancient and unchanging moral core of the doctor-patient relationship, comes an awareness of the multiple systems that influence this primary dyad, and an appreciation of just how profoundly influencing these systems are. This awareness is exemplified by the ACGME's competency in systems-based practice. After centuries, attention on protecting patients from potential abuse by physicians has expanded to include attention to protecting patients from the potential abuse of today's healthcare delivery systems.

THE TASK

The ACGME has set a difficult task for residents and resident education program directors and supervisors. The ACGME General Competency states, "The residency program must require its residents to develop the competencies in the six areas below to the level expected of a new practitioner. Toward this end, programs must define the specific knowledge, skills, and attitudes required and provide educational experiences as needed in order for their residents to demonstrate the competencies." Specific to the competency on systems-based practice, it states:

> Residents must demonstrate an awareness of and responsiveness to the larger context and system of health care and the ability to effectively call on system resources to provide care that is of optimal value. Residents are expected to:
>
> - understand how their patient care and other professional practices affect other health care professionals, the health care organization, and the larger society and how these elements of the system affect their own practice
> - know how types of medical practice and delivery systems differ from one another, including methods controlling health care costs and allocating resources
> - practice cost-effective health care and resource allocation that does not compromise quality of care
> - advocate for quality patient care and assist patients in dealing with system complexities
> - know how to partner with health care managers and health care providers to assess, coordinate, and improve health care and know how these activities can affect system performance[4]

Acquiring the requisite knowledge, skills, and attitudes will be challenging for residents. But what is interesting, and perhaps more pronounced for this competency than for any of the other five, is that assuring that residents have the educational experiences necessary to develop the knowledge, skills, and attitudes to demonstrate competency in systems-based practice will require that everyone throughout the systems in which the residents train and work model the practice of medicine with a systems-based approach. Anything less won't work.

Resident training programs are subsystems within the suprasystems in which residents work and train. No training program, whether it is of residents or any other category of trainee, will ever be successful if those who train do not model the behaviors desired of trainees. When instructors and supervisors espouse one kind of behavior but model something much less, the integrity gap is clear. This disconnection between word and deed produces cynicism in trainees, a grave outcome in young physicians. Almost 20 years ago, Donald Kanter and Philip Mervis, in their research on cynicism, found,

> Cynical tendencies are growing into a consensus world view with implications for society, commerce, and the workplace ... the cynic ... sees selfishness and fakery at the core of human nature.... Cynics mistrust ... most authority figures, regard the average person as false-faced and uncaring, and conclude that you should basically look out for yourself.... Cynics at work deeply doubt the truth of what their managements tell them and believe that ... given a chance, will take advantage of them.[5]

This sorry trend has only continued to deepen within medicine and society over the past 20 years.

That the ACGME now requires resident training that includes systems-based competencies promises that this trend may be reversed. We have the knowledge to make our healthcare systems patient-centered environments in which personnel can work together in personally and professionally rewarding ways, while, simultaneously, providing healthcare services at the highest levels of professionalism. But to achieve this possibility means our healthcare delivery operations must be totally re-engineered.

The new century has seen systems thinking move to center stage in healthcare. The Institute of Medicine (IOM) has made clear that healthcare systems must move from a self-identity as mechanical organizations to networks of complex adaptive systems (CAS).[6] This transformation requires that healthcare organizations must shift from outmoded mechanical behaviors to current systems processes. Mechanical systems are predictable and programmable; complex adaptive systems are not. Mechanical systems are composed of standardized and replicable parts; complex adaptive systems are not. Mechanical systems are characterized by ever-increasing levels of specification. Intense levels of specification will strangle and paralyze a CAS. A complex adaptive system is one that flourishes under conditions of fluid exchange of information, transparency of process and decision making, elimination of counterproductive routines, and a gentle regulatory yoke.

For residents to learn to demonstrate systems-based practice, the practices of the institutions in which they work and train must be systems-based. Because residents cannot be responsible for altering their institutional environments, it will be up to the resident education program chiefs to assure that the environment changes so that the needed educational experiences can be provided. In sum, to teach systems-based practice, a healthcare organization must become a systems-based organization. Personnel at all levels, especially those in leadership positions, must incorporate the characteristics of a CAS into their normal work patterns. That means everyone in the organization must become comfortable with change. Rules need to be simplified and their ubiquity pruned. Personnel at all systems levels need to take responsibility for actions in an environment of fewer rules and less behavioral specification. Everyone must learn to celebrate and reward novel thinking, creative problem-solving, and the discussion and disagreement required to achieve these ends. Personnel must embrace the difference between order and control, developing confidence that order, where and when needed, will emerge so that outmoded attempts at centralized, bureaucratic control can be jettisoned.

These activities are ordinarily anathema to an organization. Organizational psychology teaches that organizations, like individuals, seek stability, will squeeze out disruptive influences, and will endeavor mightily to retain the status quo. Routines are comforting to individuals and institutions. Change-agents are upsetting. But if the IOM and progressive business pundits are correct, it is just these tendencies that must be overcome if we are to train residents to become physicians practicing at the highest levels of excellence and professionalism.

Impeding this process is that the qualities of a change agent — that is, being a collaborative questioner and someone who disagrees agreeably — is not primarily the kind of skill for which physicians, especially medical students and physicians in training, have been rewarded. Rather, knowledge-based skills have been emphasized. Mastering scientific and clinical knowledge, the core skills of the medically competent physician, are not the skills considered primary for mastery of systems-based practice. Skill in systems-based practice requires mastery of complex psychological responses and the ability to engage in refined yet vigorous ethical debate. Consider the following case.

North Central Hospital's ethics committee includes two third-year residents. During an ethics committee discussion of a particularly complicated case, one of the residents disagrees with the position taken by the new chief of medicine. The chief of medicine dismisses the resident's comments, with an edge in his voice, saying that the resident is too inexperienced to understand the ethics of the case. The chairperson of the ethics committee says nothing. Nobody else gives the resident's position fair consideration. For the rest of both residents' terms on the committee, they no longer offer their opinions. Having heard the story many times over, future residents do not offer comments when the chief of medicine is present, nor do many residents call the ethics committee chairperson for consultations.

The inability of the hospital's leaders to master their psychological defenses and fears will have been a toxic lesson for the residents.

Learning to be comfortable with, or at least to tolerate, the vigorous debate called for by the medico-moral decisions clinicians and healthcare administrators make daily is a psychological skill. Regular and searing self-examination, at the individual and systems level, requires control of one's emotional defenses. Learning to challenge each other across peer groups and up, down, and across the various chains of command in ways that produce learning and collegiality takes emotional maturity. The quality of decisions that physicians make in treatment recommendations, advocacy, and resource allocation policy is based on skill in managing their own psychological responses and refinement in ethical analysis. In sum, demonstration of the ACGME systems-based practice competency outcomes will spring less from knowledge and more from mastery of ego challenge and refinement of moral judgment and debate skills.

To achieve these outcomes, healthcare environments in which residents train and practice will need to be re-engineered into settings that habituate and reward the desired behavioral outcomes. To create such environments at both the sub- and suprasystems levels, we need to turn our healthcare organizations into healthcare delivery CAS. To achieve this transformation, the reward systems in the organization need to reinforce CAS-oriented, rather than mechanical, behavior.

It is this author's hypothesis that the only way to succeed in such organizational transformation is to create morally safe environments. Only morally safe environments will create the context necessary to convert our mechanical systems into the complex adaptive systems that promise greater safety, better care for patients, and the resident competencies called for by the ACGME.

CREATING A CAS-CONDUCIVE ENVIRONMENT: THE TRICKLE DOWN, UP, ACROSS, AND THROUGH MODEL

Although physicians and others within traditional, mechanical healthcare organizations have been rewarded for adhering to mechanical behavior patterns, it is important to remember that humans can change their behavior. One of the great beauties of being human is that we can change and adapt to new information. Emotional and psychological insights can result in shifts in behavioral patterns. Evolution in ethical thinking can result in changes, for the better, in how humans treat each other, other creatures, and the environment. In short, we are learning animals.

Optimal learning occurs when an environment is designed to allow those in it to maximize their own tendencies toward critical thinking and mastery of the principles and skills being taught. In healthcare, the appropriate principles and skills are generally consistent across systems, at all sub- and suprasystem levels. These common principles and skills are summarized in the executive summary of the final report of the President's Advisory Commission on Consumer Protection and Quality in the Health Care Industry. This report states, "The purpose of the health care system must be to continually reduce the burden of illness, injury, and disability, and to improve health and functioning of the people of the United States."[7] The IOM has translated the President's Advisory Commission's broad mandate into the six specific aims that healthcare should be safe, effective, patient-centered, timely, efficient, and equitable. These aims, however, are not new. They are the same aims that have been at the heart of medicine since time immemorial.[8]

The difficulty is not in setting appropriate goals, but in how to achieve them. Given that our healthcare delivery systems are in crisis, and have been for years, mainstream thinking has just not yet identified the fundamental sources of the problems or the avenues to their solutions. But these answers already exist.

We must recognize that the problems and the solutions, at their core, are not merely technical, economic, regulatory, or informational, but ethical. Lester Thurow had this insight almost 20 years ago when he noted, "Health-care costs are being treated as if they were largely an economic problem, but they are not. To be solved, they will have to be treated as an ethical problem."[9] What Thurow understood, but what mainstream medicine has yet to appreciate, is that resolution of virtually every issue, question, or situation in medicine, whether ostensibly technical, economic, legal, regulatory, or informational, requires a moral judgment. For example, although there is no debate about whether or not informed consent documents are required for surgical procedures, it is a moral judgment about how much information is the right amount to be included. We must appreciate that decisions about what we do and how we do it always include an ethical component.

It is now time, also, to act on the insight that to solve the crisis in medicine means we must focus on the ethical climates of our healthcare organizations. We must design systems to function in ways that increase the prospect that residents, other clinicians, staff, and administrators can perform at the highest levels of professionalism. Central to the problems, and the solutions, of today's healthcare delivery systems are the ethical climates of these systems. When we take seriously that creating morally safe healthcare environments is necessary, role models can teach residents how to successfully navigate through the technical, economic, legal, regulatory, informational, and other interconnecting and interdependent systems that affect their relationships with their patients. In short, what is required is to assure that the systems in which residents work and train are morally safe environments.

THE MORALLY SAFE ENVIRONMENT

A morally safe environment is one in which all members of the organization feel safe enough to speak up. A morally safe environment is one in which all are encouraged to challenge each other about medical, economic, policy, scientific, administrative, regulatory, and ethical issues, that is, about every aspect of the functioning of all the sub- and suprasystems within and outside the organization. Creative problem-solving, willingness to admit error, openness to questioning, and change flourish in environments where these behaviors are rewarded and celebrated. Such behaviors wither away in environments that are overly controlled by hierarchy and regulatory minutia. When personal initiative and responsibility are positively reinforced, these behaviors multiply across the various organizational systems, and residents learn these skills through observation. Personal initiative and responsibility are suffocated by unnecessary lines of authority, lack of support, and heavy-handed interpretation of regulatory guidance. Under such conditions, residents become morally and intellectually paralyzed.

A morally safe environment is one in which all members of the organization feel safe enough to speak up. A training program that can teach young physicians systems-based practice requires an organization that is unthreatened by residents and others who speak up. To have residents who speak up requires that everyone in the organization feels safe. Speaking up means being comfortable asking a question or disagreeing. A morally safe environment is one in which anyone feels comfortable enough to ask anyone else a question.

Most residents have had the following experience.

> On rounds, the resident presents his/her patient, having already had a lengthy conversation with fellow residents about the patient's care. The attending orders a test or initiates a treatment that had already been considered and rejected by the residents, yet nobody speaks up. None of the involved residents challenge the attending or even asks why he or she is ordering the test or treatment. Nobody says anything because the moral courage needed is absent.

Direct interchange between residents and more senior physicians, however, is only one subsystem in which the morally safe environment needs to be created. Systems thinking requires that residents and others learn to appreciate how systems are intertwined. The systems of physician and nurse, or physician and social worker, are other examples of where individual behavior will have large spill-over effects on residents' learning. In a CAS, these subsystems will be open to rigorous discussion, hearty disagreement, and transparency in decision making. In so doing, patients' well-being, staff's satisfaction, and respectful clinical relationships can be maximized. Take the following scenario.

Mrs. G is an 85-year-old patient with metastatic colon cancer and multiple co-morbidities who is minimally responsive. The patient's adult son is questioning the nurses and social worker whether or not his mother has gone through enough curative treatment attempts. Mrs. G's oncologist, however, cuts the son off and won't discuss the matter with the nurses or social worker. Instead, the physician paints a positive picture to the son about the length of potential life left and says that if they insert a feeding tube, Mrs. G can gain strength and live for many more months, if not longer. After several failed attempts to discuss the matter with the physician, the social worker calls an ethics committee consultation. When the physician hears of the consult he is incensed, threatening to have the social worker fired.

This case is a prime example of everything that is wrong with traditional medical practice. Today, such behavior has a name: *rankism*, or *rank-based abuse*. A term recently coined by Robert Fuller, rankism "is the 'cancer' that underlies many of the seemingly disparate maladies that afflict the body politic. The outrage over self-serving corrupt executives is indignation over rankism. Sexual abuse by clergy is rankism. Elder abuse in life care facilities is rankism. Scientists taking credit for their assistants' research is rankism,"[10] and physicians riding rough-shod over surrogates, nurses, and social workers is rankism. Although such behavior is obviously unacceptable, it happens all the time. Resident education program directors and supervisors have the obligation to prevent others from polluting the moral climate of the organization. The organization's response will have important implications for systems' functioning and will dictate what residents learn.

If Mrs. G's physician admits large numbers of patients, the hospital may be disinclined to rein in his bad behavior. But not doing so will have serious repercussions. Nurses and social workers throughout the organization will be intimidated and angry, psychological states that predispose clinicians to burnout. The residents will learn that, if not acceptable, it is tolerable for at least some physicians, most notably high admitting physicians, to get away with bad behavior. This information is a recipe for cynicism.

If, on the other hand, the ethics committee consultation results in a formal rebuke of the physician and a clear explanation that such behavior will not be tolerated, everyone's inclination to speak up will have been strengthened. Residents will have had the appropriate behaviors modeled for them. Both the requirement to challenge their peers who act badly and proper interactions among physicians, staff, and family members will be clarified. And, consistent with the CAS characteristic of nonlinearity, it would not be surprising to find that the hospital that responds this way has fewer nursing vacancies than surrounding facilities.

CREATING A MORALLY SAFE ENVIRONMENT

Creating a morally safe environment is a long-term venture. Creating systems in which any relevantly involved individual feels comfortable enough to speak up takes care, time, and attention. Speaking up isn't easy. It takes moral courage. Fortunately, moral courage is a virtue we can learn.

From Aristotle to B.F. Skinner to more contemporary authors, it seems clear that moral courage, and its manifestation of comfort in speaking up, can be learned. What is clear, also, is that conditions need to be right to allow the requisite learning to take place. In Aristotelian terms, the process goes as follows: "of all the things that come to us by nature we first acquire the potentiality and later exhibit the activity (this is plain in the case of the senses . . .) but the virtues we get by first exercising them. . . . For the things we have to learn before we can do them, we learn by doing them, e.g. men become builders by building and lyre players by playing the lyre; so too we become just by doing just acts, temperate by doing temperate acts, brave by doing brave acts."[11] The implications for systems-based practice, if true, are substantial. Physicians who threaten social workers produce residents who habituate into senior attendings who threaten social workers. Physicians who respect the views of social workers and see ethics consultations as opportunities for expanded moral analysis produce residents who do as well. This Aristotelian notion that doing the good produces skill in figuring out what the good is and doing it again might seem like philosophical wishful thinking, were it not for modern scientific validation.

Classic Skinnerian theory teaches that individuals are inclined to repeat behaviors for which they have been rewarded. The mountains of data that support this theory show us that if persons are rewarded for doing the good, they are, as Aristotle predicted, inclined toward doing so again and again. Skinner extends this insight into the realm of group influences on individual behavior: "In a given instance, good behavior on the part of A may be positively reinforced by B because it generates an emotional disposition on the part of B to 'do good' to A . . . it seems clear, simply as a matter of observation, that the behavior of favoring another is modified by appropriate emotional circumstances and that good behavior on the part of another is a case in point."[12]

In turn, Skinner's hypotheses about environmental influences on individual behavior have been supported by more recent research. Synthesizing a body of research studying cognitive bias in human interaction, Robert H. Frank summarizes, "Once the initial valence has been assigned, a biased cognitive filter becomes activated. You still evaluate further aspects of your experience with a new acquaintance, but with a slant. If the initial evaluation was positive, you are much more likely to treat ambiguous signals in a positive light. But if your initial impression was negative, you are more likely to assign negative interpretations to those same signals."[13] In healthcare, in which the mission is other-oriented, it is critically important that the environmental stimuli produce behaviors that reinforce other-oriented behavior, be it toward patients, surrogates, colleagues, or others.

Let us consider the case in which one of the "others" in a healthcare organization felt safe enough to speak up, to appreciate how important this issue is for systems-based practice.

At a large research center, there was a long-term study of young adult patient-subjects with a chronic pain syndrome. Many of these subjects had been on the study since their early teens. Study procedures required that subjects come into the research facility once a year for a three-week period. Over the years of study participation, the subjects had developed very close relationships with the principle investigator (PI), who, since the beginning of the study many years before, had risen from fellow through the ranks to department chairperson. The PI was a highly private person by temperament and not easily approachable by junior members of the research team.

During the stay of a particular subject, one of the housekeeping staff noticed that the subject was out of his room more often than the other subjects. Paying closer attention, this housekeeper watched the subject enter the elevators with undue frequency. Finally, the housekeeper got on the elevator when the subject and a visitor got on the elevator together. During the elevator ride, the housekeeper observed the friend injecting something into the subject's venous access.

When the housekeeper reported it to one of the research fellows on the protocol, she was told not to get involved, that the fellow would handle it. But the situation continued. Mustering what must have been significant moral courage, she reported the incident to one of the nurses, who then brought the problem to the appropriate staff. It was determined that the subject's friend was injecting illicit drugs into the subject, and a sitter was attached to the subject for the rest of his stay.

In some facilities, a housekeeper might be considered too insignificant to a patient or subject's direct care to have any important information to provide. When such an individual has information that challenges the status quo, a traditionally hierarchical, mechanical organization will be prone to dismiss the housekeeper's report. In a CAS, however, one understands that no system is completely detached from any other, and rankism is flattened, when appropriate, to surfacing problems. In a morally safe environment, it is appreciated that nobody in the organization has any greater moral authority than anyone else for illuminating and resolving a problem. Fortunately for subjects' safety, this facility had created an environment in which all individuals felt responsible for the well-being of the subjects.

The following case demonstrates the opposite; that is, how inappropriate application of power withers moral courage.

In a large university medical center, a problem had been identified in the review and oversight of a prominent researcher's work. Briefly, it was alleged that a PI (principle investigation), who was also a department chairperson, had engaged in research on tissue samples, appropriately obtained for one purpose, without approval by the institutional review board (IRB), for another purpose. In a special meeting of the IRB, a junior investigator challenged the PI about his actions. When the meeting ended, the PI stormed directly into the office of the IRB member's department chairperson, demanding that the junior investigator be removed from the IRB.

The department chairperson had several projects in which his own work, and that of his laboratory, was dependent on the collaboration and good will of the PI. After the PI stormed back out of the office, the department chairperson went to the junior investigator and suggested that perhaps she might have served on the IRB long enough and that she might want to step off the committee. The department chairperson didn't order the junior investigator to step off, nor did he make the suggestion in an angry tone of voice. Neither was necessary to produce a chilling effect on everyone in the department.

BUILDING THE CRITICAL MASS TO SUSTAIN A MORALLY SAFE ENVIRONMENT

As easy as it is to have one or two persons pollute the moral climate, the reverse seems not to apply. It is not enough to have one or even a few individuals within the organization known as wise counselors. The change needed to move an organization from a mechanical system to a CAS, to produce residents who are skilled at systems-based practice, to create the necessary morally safe environments, requires a critical mass of ethically sensitive persons throughout the organization. As Fuller notes, "Typically, psychological change precedes a political assault on the status quo. Not until a great many individuals conclude that something is wrong and that an alternative exists will they organize politically and try to bring down an existing edifice."[14] A few "high visibility" good souls will never have the influence, energy, authority, and emotional strength needed to change organizational culture.

Rather, what is needed is a critical mass of ethics-focused individuals within and across the multiple systems of the organization. Starting from the top down, the organization needs persons who are identifiable as ethically thoughtful and interested, throughout all sectors. Such persons initiate discussion about the ethical implications of issues, as they arise, throughout daily work. They encourage and model thoughtful ethical discussion. They are comfortable with, and engage in, disagreements agreeably. Such individuals act as magnets for all of the rest of the persons within their normal daily venues who are also interested in ethical issues, but may not have quite as much psychological strength. These others may not be the ones to expose the ethical aspects of a complex issue, initiate discussions, or openly start a disagreement, but they will join the process if given encouragement by those they know and trust. This is how moral courage is learned, and how the necessary critical mass of ethics-focused persons develops. Once there are enough of these persons, when issues have to be handled across multiple other systems, there will be enough persons within all of the systems that the characteristics of a CAS can flourish.

One source for producing this critical mass is through a vibrant and highly functioning ethics committee. Consider a slightly altered version of the first case presented in this chapter.

North Central Hospital's ethics committee includes two third-year residents. During an ethics committee discussion of a particularly complicated case, one of the residents disagrees with the position taken by the new chief of medicine. The chief of medicine, in a neutral tone of voice, says he really thinks his position is the ethically optimal solution and gives his reasons. The ethics committee chairperson, agreeing that the chief's position is sound, nonetheless takes over the argumentation process from the resident. He then shapes the resident's position into a quite elegant and ethically acceptable option. After that, the chair invites the rest of the committee to think through the two positions as potential boundaries of ethically acceptable possibilities, challenging the other committee members to offer up their own positions, either novel to the two on the table, or elaborations of either one. Lively and substantive ethical analysis ensues. The committee ultimately comes to a consensus that favors the essence of the chief's position, but includes nuances that only surfaced as a result of the additional considerations raised by the resident and others on the committee.

For the rest of both residents' terms on the committee, they participate thoughtfully in committee discussions and promote the committee to the junior residents who will take their places. The chairperson of the ethics committee begins to notice an increase in "curb-sides" and formal consultations coming from the residents across various units in the hospital.

Word spreads quickly among residents that neither one was "shut down" by the chief of medicine in a meeting, or that, in a disagreement with the chief of medicine, the ethics committee chairperson brought an evenhandedness to the situation that made everyone more comfortable.

The quality of nonlinearity is, as the IOM noted, "Small changes can have large effects; a large program in an organization might have little actual impact, yet a rumor could touch off a union organizing effort."[15] How such a situation is handled will have a ripple effect throughout the organization that can be expected to increase or decrease residents' psychological ability to speak up.

But even having a superior ethics committee is not going to be enough. What is needed is a critical mass of individuals, strategically located across multiple systems, who are committed to focusing on ethics. Further, it is important that these individuals are at the highest levels of leadership across all systems of the organization. As Christopher Meyers states, "Organizational culture is created and maintained by two processes: the top-down establishment of institutional values by owners and managers and the carrying out of those values by in-the-trenches employees."[16] Ethics is the art of persuasion. Moral judgments are only forceful if those who offer them are viewed as wise, respected individuals. Because ethical recommendations lack the force of law, strong intellectual, political, and psychological levers are required to move heavy behavioral objects. That is, when moral judgment faces long-standing practices, it takes great moral force to produce a shift. This moral force is generated by a growing, and highly visible, group of individuals within an organization who actively participate within their own systems-based practices to advance the creation and maintenance of a morally safe environment. Everyone from the top down encourages and rewards others for speaking up, and takes a firm hand in retraining, or eliminating, those who do not.

REDUCING THE WEIGHT OF REGULATION

Efforts to create and maintain an ethical climate will also require reducing the weight of regulatory and legal ways of thinking. Charity Scott notes, "Law pervades medicine because ethics pervades medicine, and in America, we use the law to resolve ethical dilemmas in health care."[17] But this process stifles ability to engage in ethically sensitive systems behavior and is a threat to the well-being of patients. Psychologically, excessive reliance on regulation and compliance may merely be place markers for fear of litigation. Excessive fear of litigation can obliterate individual common sense, self-reliance, creative problem-solving, and ethical behavior, a point already long appreciated.[18] When excessive fear of litigation produces overly legalistic regulatory interpretations and conflates ethics with compliance, the ability of a CAS to overcome mechanical behavior is doomed.

Regulations and compliance are necessary and important. It is, however, the way in which an organization interprets regulations and implements compliance programs that will set the tone for individual and systems behaviors. There can be little that is more mechanical than excessively legalistic thinking. Where it exists, it permeates not merely those who have direct responsibility for regulatory oversight and compliance, but everyone in the organization. Worst of all, such thinking leaves physicians intellectually paralyzed and ethically confused. Modeling such behavior for residents may be lethal to their ability to mature into senior physicians who exemplify the qualities identified by the IOM as critical to improved patient care and safety.[19] This does not suggest that we should deregulate our healthcare organizations or weaken our insistence on legal compliance. What it means is that we must begin to shape our interpretations of legal and regulatory matters within a framework that focuses on their ethical basis.

To achieve this revolution in legal thinking and regulatory implementation, an ethical approach must be taken to deciding what is necessary. An ethical approach to regulatory compliance and legal interpretation calls on all who must comply with laws and regulations — that is, everyone — to think through how they comply. Asking what the ethically optimal way to interpret and comply with the law or regulation must be the framework for analysis. In a healthcare organization, that means asking such questions as, "What would be in the best interest of this patient?" "What is the organization's obligation to the patient, surrogate, nurse, social worker, et cetera?" "What does justice, fairness, and/or common decency suggest is owed to the patient, surrogate, nurse, social worker, et cetera?" Once consensus around these answers is determined, we can think through how the answers might be consistent or inconsistent with legal and regulatory interpretations.

At their finest, laws and regulations set minimal behavioral standards that are sufficiently elastic to allow for maturing interpretation as the moral norms on which they are based evolve. Such excellence in regulatory guidance is exemplified by the regulations governing the ethical conduct of publicly funded human subjects research in the United States.[20] These regulations are brief — barely 20 pages — and have been revised infrequently and minimally since they were promulgated two decades ago. During this period, ethical debate in the professional and lay literature about the ethically appropriate conduct of human subjects research has mushroomed, but these elegantly written regulations continue to be relevant. The regulations have not changed; interpretation of how they should be implemented has changed.

Contrast this example of regulatory excellence with the following.

A patient is brought into an intensive care unit (ICU) in the middle of the night in need of surgery. Upon admission he is still conscious and capacitated, and makes it clear to the medical team that he is a practicing Jehovah's Witness and does not want any blood. Shortly thereafter, he becomes unresponsive. The family members with him are not Jehovah's Witnesses. Once the patient loses decisional capacity and they are now being asked to provide procedural consents, they tell the medical team that if he needs blood they should go ahead and give it to him.

The next morning on rounds these events are discussed. The bioethicist asked the resident why nobody from the patient's Jehovah's Witness community was called to come and advocate on behalf of the patient. The resident responded that he hadn't thought of it, but wouldn't have done so anyway because it would have been a violation of HIPAA (the Health Insurance Portability and Accountability Act of 1996).[21]

A response of, "Well, let's think this through some more — HIPAA violation or eternal damnation?" resulted in laughter among the team and a look of dismayed shock and unhappy insight on the resident's part that he had made the wrong decision.

A strict HIPAA constructionist might consider contacting a member of the patient's faith community a violation, especially when the patient had caring, if perhaps ethically misguided, family members acting on his behalf. But a loose constructionist might interpret contacting the patient's spiritual leader to be acceptable under the HIPAA allowance for sharing information necessary for patient care. Further confusing the resident, however, was the ubiquitous and misguided legal interpretation about who was the appropriate decision maker. Because traditional medical practice and most surrogacy laws put family members first in line, there was no ethical analysis of whether the family members, in having given permission for a blood transfusion that was refused by the patient, were acting in an ethically, or even legally, appropriate way on the patient's behalf. The resident's fear of litigation by an angry family member inhibited his moral judgment. That nobody else suggested calling a member of the patient's faith community indicates a lack of ethical imagination.

This is a common problem in healthcare facilities in which risk management has the overly anxious and confused view that upholding patients' autonomy and obtaining informed consent means that whatever the patient or family member wants, goes. Such confusion is less likely in an institution in which risk management's contribution to creating a morally safe environment is supportive. Ethically sound risk managers make explicit that physicians are encouraged to work through the various systems of consensus building and consultation, and once all relevantly involved parties have agreed on the best course of action for the patient, risk management will support their decision, regardless of legal outcome. Legal doctrines, case law, and regulations should provide guidance and wisdom. Becoming slavishly tied to over-interpretation of laws and regulations robs residents of the ability to learn to think ethically. As Scott states,

> Law came to the patients' bedside . . . because there was an emerging societal sense that wrong was being done to the patients there. This invitation to get the law involved in ethical conflicts is nothing new. Whenever there is a social sense of wrong, or injustice, or an abuse of power by some people or some institutions . . . those who feel abused often turn to the law for protection . . . a felt need for patient protection from a power imbalance in the doctor-patient relationship has resulted in consent forms, living wills, and other legal documents and rules. That these legal mechanisms frequently provide only minimal protections in practice — that they often fail to achieve the ethical balance that was their goal — does not alter the point that their purpose was to promote an ethical vision of the doctor-patient relationship. . . . And herein lies the pitfall which the very power of the law creates for ethical reflection. . . . Law only sets a floor for ethical behavior. . . . Faced with the power of law, however, we tend

to get stuck in our ethical reflections at the ground floor. As is so often true when law packs ethics with a punch, people tend to over-focus on avoiding the punch, and not on the ethical underpinnings of the law.[22]

For residents to reach the highest levels of professionalism, they must have models who interpret laws and regulations to maximize patient care, not in ways that some might think will avoid the punch of litigations. Overly legalistic interpretation does not prevent litigation, only the ethical practice of medicine protects against litigation.[23] This is a lesson residents must learn and that can only be taught in healthcare organizations that have adopted an ethical approach to legal and regulatory interpretation.

CONCLUSIONS

Why is the ACGME competency in systems-based practice so important? It originates with the ancient principles that define the ethical conduct of medicine — act in the patient's best interest and protect patients from harm. The ascendancy of the autonomy movement was a way of protecting patients from the tyranny of medical paternalism. Having young physicians learn how to think not only on an individual level, but also at a systems level, is a way to protect patients from the tyranny of systems. Take, for example, advance directives. Advance directives can be thought of as a systems issue. At the supra-systems level, there is a federal law requiring hospitals and other healthcare organizations to find out if patients have advance directives, and, if not, whether patients want information about them. At the sub-systems level, healthcare organizations spend inordinate amounts of time figuring out how to implement the federal law, how to demonstrate to the Joint Commission on Accreditation of Healthcare Organizations (JCAHO) that the law is implemented, determining which staff will have responsibility for which parts of the process, and designing advance directive information to be provided to patients. All this effort and the following still happens.

Mrs. Jones is going into surgery to repair a broken hip. Her only relative, her granddaughter, has been with her since she arrived at the hospital two days ago. Although Mrs. Jones lives alone, her granddaughter is her only relative. They have always been so close that

Mrs. Jones has a durable power of attorney for person and property, including healthcare decisions, naming the granddaughter as her agent. In all the commotion, the granddaughter has only now produced the documentation. Mrs. Jones is sedated and prepped for surgery. The nurse looks over the document before putting it on the chart and sees that it says, ". . . only in the state of Michigan." The patient is in Illinois.

This jurisdictional discrepancy halts the patient's surgery. The nurse calls the resident, who is unwilling to allow the patient to proceed to surgery because now the patient is thought not to have the "right" advance directive. The resident calls the surgeon, who won't operate, because the surgeon doesn't know if the paperwork is legal in the state of Illinois. The surgeon calls the hospital's risk management department, who then calls hospital counsel. Hospital counsel takes several hours to decide that an advance directive executed in Michigan can be used in Illinois. By this time, the patient's surgery has to be put off until the next day, causing distress to the patient and granddaughter and wasting operating room resources.

If an ethics approach had been taken, the scenario might have gone more like the following.

The nurse realizes that the documentation is legally authorized only in Michigan and reports the matter to the resident. The resident, who is comfortable questioning what systems approach might be best implemented to handle this question, decides to check with a peer who sits on the hospital's ethics committee. That resident explains that all that is required to be an ethically and legally valid surrogate is, in the absence of documented agency, that the person acting as surrogate appears to be acting in the best interest of the patient. It doesn't matter whether or not Illinois considers the Michigan document a legal assignment of agency. If the granddaughter is the ethically appropriate surrogate, this meets every ethical and legal principle upon which the suprasystem of advance directives sits. The resident responsible for the patient's care then calls the surgeon, explains the situation, and makes the recommendation that the granddaughter is the appropriate surrogate. The patient then moves on to her surgery as planned.

Wasting resources, provoking anxiety and frustration in patients and surrogates, and putting patients at risk from process errors are harmful outcomes that can be avoided through skillful systems-based practice. Avoiding such outcomes, however, does not mean that such problems can ever be eradicated completely. The systems in which residents work and train are so complex that errors and problems will always occur. The hope is not for perfection, but rather for the creation of environments that present the greatest opportunities for medical excellence. The promise that such environments will become the norm rather than the exception is on the horizon. Organizations such as the Institute for Health Care Improvement (*www.ihi.org*) have been created to assist in this process. For resident training, environments are required that reward the psychological responses and ethical discussions necessary for superior patient care. Now it is up to those responsible for resident training programs to create the morally safe environments necessary to assure that the residents they train can demonstrate the ACGME-required performance outcomes in systems-based practice.

ACKNOWLEDGMENTS

The author wishes to thank Jack Lynch, MD, Center for Ethics, Washington Hospital Center, Washington, D.C.; Jonathan Moreno, PhD, Kornfield Professor of Biomedical Ethics and Director, Center for Biomedical Ethics, University of Virginia, Charlottesville, Virginia; and Jack Schwartz, JD, Assistant Attorney General and Director for Health Policy Development at the Office of the Maryland Attorney General, Baltimore, Maryland, for their review and comments on an early draft of this manuscript, and to Elizabeth Griffin, Falmouth, Massachusetts, for her excellent copy editing.

An earlier version of this chapter appeared in *Organizational Ethics: Healthcare, Business, and Policy*, volume 2, no.1 (Spring 2005). ©2005, University Publishing Group. Used with permission. All rights reserved.

NOTES

1. Accreditation Council for Graduate Medical Education, *www.acgme.org/outcome/comp/compFull.asp* or see the appendix in this volume.
2. R.D. Stacey, *Strategic Management and Organizational Dynamics: The Challenge of Complexity* (New York: Prentice-Hall, 2003).

3. Versipan Study, *http://www.ihc.com/xp/ihc/aboutihc/news/article8.xml.*
4. ACGME, see note 1 above.
5. D.L. Kanter and P.H. Mirvis, *The Cynical Americans: Living and Working in an Age of Discontent and Dissillusion* (San Francisco, Calif.: Jossey-Bass, 1989), 2.
6. Institute of Medicine, *Crossing the Quality Chasm: A New Health System for the 21st Century* (Washington, D.C.: National Academy Press, 2001).
7. President's Advisory Commission on Consumer Protection and Quality in the Health Care Industry, *Quality First: Better Health Care for All Americans, http://www.hcqualitycommission.gov/final/execsum.html,* accessed 8 January 2005.
8. IOM, see note 6 above.
9. L.C. Thurow, "Learning to Say 'No'," *New England Journal of Medicine* 311, no. 24 (1984): 1569-72, p. 1572.
10. R.W. Fuller, *Somebodies and Nobodies: Overcoming the Abuse of Rank* (Gabriola Island, B.C., Canada: New Society Publishers, 2003), 3.
11. Aristotle, *The Nicomachean Ethics,* trans. D. Ross and rev. J.L. Ackrill and U.O. Urmson (New York: Oxford University Press, 1998), 28-9.
12. B.F. Skinner, *Science and Human Behavior* (New York: Free Press, 1965), 325.
13. R.H. Frank, *What Price the Moral High Ground? Ethical Dilemmas in Competitive Environments* (Princeton, N.J.: Princeton University Press, 2004), 15.
14. Fuller, see note 10 above, p. 61.
15. IOM, see note 6 above.
16. C. Meyers, "Institutional Culture and Individual Behavior: Creating an Ethical Environment," *Science and Engineering Ethics* 10, no. 2 (2004): 269-76.
17. C. Scott, "Why Law Pervades Medicine: An Essay on Ethics in Health Care," *Notre Dame Journal of Law, Ethics, & Public Policy* 14, no. 1(2000): 245-303, p. 302.
18. P.K. Howard, *Death of Common Sense: How Law Is Suffocating America* (New York: Warner Books, 2001).
19. IOM, see note 6 above.
20. U.S. Department of Health and Human Services, National Institutes of Health, and Office for Human Research Protections, "The Common Rule," Title 45 (Public Welfare), *Code of Federal Regulations,* Part 46 (Protection of Human Subjects) (Washing-

ton, D.C.: DHHS, revised 13 November 2001; effective 13 December 2001).

21. Health Insurance Portability and Accountability Act of 1996, *http://www.hhs.gov/ocr/hipaa/finalreg.html*.

22. Scott, see note 17 above, p. 12-13.

23. H. Forster, J. Schwartz, and E.G. DeRenzo, "How to Reduce Legal Risk and Improve Patient Satisfaction," *Archives of Internal Medicine* 162, no. 11 (2002): 1217-9; R. Anand, J. Schwartz, and E.G. DeRenzo, "True Risk Management: Physicians' Liability Risk and the Practice of Patient-Centered Medicine," *Journal of Law and Health* (in press).

Learning and Growth

8

Professionalism, Humanism, Mindfulness, and the Healthcare Melee

Daniel M. Becker and Matthew J. Goodman

> *It is the humdrum, day-in, day-out, everyday work that is the real satisfaction of the practice of medicine. . . .* — William Carlos Williams

INTRODUCTION

Picture this: two physicians share a small office in a busy university-based general medicine practice. They listen to the other's dictations, conversations with house staff, requests for consultations, bargains with utilization review, appeals for non-formulary prescriptions, justifications for MRIs, excuses (often lame) to spouses and children waiting at home, swaps for nights and weekends on-call, tart answers to nurses who need to squeeze someone else into a fully booked schedule. They are earnest, well-trained, diligent, caring, experienced, and human. They trade war stories and remember the days of the giants, every third night on-call, every other night in the ICU. They trade coding tips. Without envy or pride they compare their running tally of RVUs (relative value units). It turns out they are equally unproductive, but improving, staying out of trouble. They mention novels, poems, music, and movies they think the other should read or see or listen to. They forward e-mail with politically incorrect jokes. For days and weeks the younger one comes to work, and, first thing in the morning, calls the same patient, a woman with a chronic illness, a broken family, a downward spiral; shame, guilt, anger, loss, and pain (there are five, not just four, horsemen of medical apocalypse), more pain than she can bear. He listens carefully and after a while will say something like, "I know that must be terrible." His older colleague stops what he is doing to follow the conversation, as if turning on a soap opera, life imitating bad art. "Can you believe it?" they ask one another afterward. They can, day after incredulous day.

The medical profession is curious, introspective, ambitious, and embattled. The high-minded behaviors and attributes that imbue clinical science with compassion and justice must not only make sense to a skeptical public, but also in a marketplace that is indifferent to the art of medicine. It still takes seven years, after college, to become a general internist or pediatrician or family physician. But every year there is more to know; more patients to see in a shorter time; more rules for billing, documentation, and credentialing; more insurance barriers that limit access to new medications, treatments, and tests; more questions from patients who now inform and misinform themselves on the internet; more complicated patients as the population ages and people survive past 80 despite chronic illness; more choice as complementary medical disciplines compete with allopathic practitioners; more layers in the healthcare sandwich; more angst in the age of terrorism.

Patients seem to expect more from their doctor. Health systems expect more because they need more. Organized medicine, in an alphabet chorus (ACP-ASIM, EFIM, AAMC, and ACGME), have spelled it out (see table 8.1).[1]

Loyal, honest, brave, clean, et cetera; fortunately, virtue is its own reward. Many doctors were Eagle Scouts even before becoming doctors. The question is not whether these expectations are fair or unfair. The first lesson of doctoring, as in parenting, is that life isn't fair. The question is how: how to maintain a sense of purpose and direction in the cross currents of complicated illness, evolving practice standards, growing liability threats, shrinking resources; how to teach medical students and residents to be compassionate as well as technologically proficient; how to maintain the commitment to patients without paying too high a personal price; how to cherish the privilege of being with patients during the worst moments of lives too short or too long; how to remain curious and involved, but, like quicksand, not too involved.

How can doctors, in training and in practice, not only survive but thrive? This essay attempts a three-part answer while raising only the important rhetorical questions. First, we will consider the central dilemma of medical practice in the twenty-first century. How to do more with less? Doctors are busier than ever. Patients are more informed than ever, and, as a consequence, expect more. Second, we will offer a few partial solutions, acknowledging that dilemmas are not supposed to be solved. In good design less is more. What does a particular patient need at a particular moment? Which details solve the clinical puzzle?

Table 8.1
The Good Physician

American Association of Medical Colleges (AAMC)[1]
- Knowledgeable (scientific method, biomedicine)
- Skillful (clinical skills, reasoning, communication, management)
- Altruistic (respect, compassion, ethics, honesty)
- Dutiful (advocacy, outreach, prevention, information management)

Accreditation Council for Graduate Medical Education (ACGME)[2]
- Medical knowledge
- Practice-based learning
- Patient care
- Interpersonal and communication skills
- Systems-based practice
- Professionalism (respect, compassion, integrity, responsiveness, altruism, ethics, commitment to excellence, cultural sensitivity)

Physician Charter: American Board of Internal Medicine, American College of Physicians, American Society of Internal Medicine, European Federation of Internal Medicine (ABIM, ACP-ASiM, EFIM)[3]
- Professionalism: foundation of the social contract for medicine
- Principles: primacy of patient welfare, patient autonomy, social justice
- Commitments to professional competence and responsibilities, confidentiality, improving quality of care, maintaining appropriate relationships, scientific knowledge, managing conflicts of interest, honesty, improving access, just distribution of finite resources

NOTES
1. *http://www.aamc.org/sitemap/start.htm.*
2. See the appendix of this volume.
3. *http://www.abinfoundation.org/pdf/ABIM_charter_lns.pdf.*

Third, we will broaden the context of the discussion and place the physician in an organization, thereby justifying the inclusion of this essay as a chapter in a book whose main concern is systems-informed professionalism. How do round pegs fit into square holes?

Three caveats: first, we are general internists, with 40 years of experience between us, and while we may indulge the conceit that we can speak for other general internists and perhaps for other primary care physicians, it is almost certain that subspecialities and hospital-based physicians face different logistical, administrative, clinical, and professional challenges. To paraphrase Tolstoy in the opening paragraph of *Anna Karenina,* all unhappy families are unhappy in unique ways. Second, for whatever reasons related to temperament, background, role models, training, literary taste, et cetera, we are interested in patients' stories and have developed the patience needed to listen closely as these stories expand and complicate over years and decades of a doctor-patient relationship. Third, we have persuaded ourselves that work and home are reciprocal endeavors. To be happy and fulfilled at work, we seek happiness and fulfillment outside work. This third caveat is free. Take it home.

MORE WITH LESS?

Recently a patient asked for a carotid ultrasound she didn't need. Someone once heard a bruit. Ever since her carotids have been silent, but she still can't stop worrying about a stroke. Her doctor had his hand on the doorknob as he briefly argued the study was not necessary. The ultrasound turned out to be normal, and Medicare wouldn't pay. The patient won't pay either, on principle. She wants the doctor to justify the test to Medicare. He is tempted to tell the truth.

• • •

An uninsured farmer drives 50 miles for his clinic visit, except he can't drive and paid a neighbor $50 to drive him. He can't drive because he can't see due to diabetes. But help is on the way. Once he starts dialysis, Medicaid and Medicare will kick in. Meanwhile, there are sample meds, and, for the doctors at noon, a free lunch, courtesy of a pharmaceutical rep.

Professionalism, Humanism, Mindfulness, and the Healthcare Melee

• • •

A man comes to clinic for a blood pressure check. He starts crying when he sees his doctor. It's a long story. The five-minute appointment lasts 30 minutes. Fortunately, if the visit is documented properly, with counseling time noted, insurance should pay. The next day the patient drops off some Family Medical Leave forms he'd like his doctor to fill out, "in his spare time, no rush, end of the week is fine."

• • •

To avoid a cut in salary, a salaried physician must meet clinical productivity goals, established prospectively and adjusted according to other sources of revenue, such as research grants or support for administrative duties. As clinical revenue increases proportionally, the productivity bar is raised. It's the converse of Zeno's paradox — the more patients seen, the more patients that need to be seen.

• • •

After five letters to the third party, authorization for gastric bypass surgery is granted. The grateful patient bakes a chocolate cake for her letter-writing doctor benefactor.

• • •

The hospital is full. The emergency room is full of patients waiting to be admitted. The ICUs are full of patients who need step-down units. The post-anesthesia unit is full of patients who had surgery and now need a room in the hospital. The community hospital downtown is full. On the general medicine service, patients can't leave because there are no nursing home beds. In clinic, a doctor reconsiders and decides that his 90-year-old patient with pneumonia is not really that sick and could be treated at home. The family thinks they are lucky their doctor makes house calls. The doctor calls the home health nurse.

Physicians are supposed to be patient advocates and to be there when needed. They are also supposed to parcel finite resources on behalf of the systems and payers that make services available. In an earlier chapter in this book and in a recent essay, Spencer and Bigoney outline the conflicts between traditional medical ethics and the expectations created by ACGME competencies that link professional ethics and business ethics.[2] The vignettes in the preceding paragraphs illustrate these conflicts and also demonstrate some of the ways physicians manage to slip out of tight spots. When push comes to shove, the doctor-patient relationship wins. Doctors do not like to say no. Patient satisfaction scores improve when gates are opened not closed, when free samples are offered, when doctors make time to listen, when battles are waged to extend benefits. If questions arise over medical benefits (the newest medication, hospitalization, a special scan, a second or third opinion in another city) physicians don't have to think very long about whom they work for, the patient or the insurance company. Most of the time it feels better to take the patient's side. Even if the customer is not always right, assuming they are saves time.

Exceptions to such beneficence can occur if the reward system is pernicious. Let's assume for the purpose of this chapter that doctors will provide care that is indicated, will think about providing care that may be indicated, will be inclined to provide care in 50:50 situations if they are rewarded for doing so (to a hammer, everything's a nail), and will not withhold care for the exclusive purpose of the year-end bonus.

Interpretations of physician advocacy should also take into account the dark cloud of medical liability. It is important to get along with patients. The good clinician wants to understand why the patient is angry. The cautious physician understands that angry patients are litigious.

From the management point of view, there is a down side to physicians as patient advocates. Physicians are tempted to game the system on behalf of their patients. They tell white lies. Uninsured patients get undercoded, easier for the salaried doctor than the public facility whose Medicaid payment may be linked to accurate coding. Supplies are given away to make it easier for patients to dress wounds or wrap sprained ankles. Sample shelves are raided and the early morning patient gets more free medicine than the late afternoon patient. Screening tests for asymptomatic patients are obtained with invented symptoms. Newer medications are obtained with embellished accounts of treatment failures using the generic formulation.

If physicians can't say no to reasonable requests, what about unreasonable requests? What about end-of-life care, treating the hopelessly ill? Again, it is easier for physicians to take one cautious step after another down the slippery slope of usual care regardless of prognosis, a path that imposes on system resources, than to have the difficult conversation, however appropriate on clinical grounds, that shifts the paradigm from cure to comfort. However, once the palliative care process begins, it is quickly embraced. It often turns out that physicians can do more with less in palliative care and hospice settings. By focusing on relief of pain or dyspnea, rather than cure, the palliative care team usually manages to relieve suffering without shortening life. Palliative and hospice care, through its emphasis on teamwork and carefully managed resources, is an important example of systems-based practice in which traditional doctor-patient ethics dovetail with organizational ethics. However, even though hospice and the referring physician share the same goal, comfort for the patient, they do not necessarily agree on the resources that should be brought to bear to achieve comfort.

Hospice care is capitated, and therefore expensive interventions such as hospitalization, radiation therapy, and/or chemotherapy for palliation, CT and MRI scanning, bone marrow growth factors, transfusions, and an array of non-generic pharmaceuticals are frowned on, if not forbidden. It is usually easy to reconcile the physician's impulse to get what's best for the patient and the hospice's instinct to survive financially. If the patient is referred to hospice at the appropriate time, and if the patient and family know what is in store, then conflicts regarding over-utilization are avoided.

The hospice and palliative model of care, putting comfort ahead of cure, could be applied to many of the chronic and incurable illnesses that compromise function in the last 10 years of life. "Hospice-lite," if you will. A further and radical reordering of priorities, focusing on comfort, prevention, and public health, while factoring out liability concerns and exaggerated faith in medical technology, would allow the U.S. healthcare system to do more with less. This is a system that spends about twice as much per capita as any other wealthy industrialized nation, and while a patient in Chicago might not have to wait long for a hip replacement, in the innercity mothers die after delivery more often than in Europe, or Japan, or Cuba.[3] Cuba! The purpose of this chapter, and the book that contains it, is not to critique the American way of life and death. Nevertheless, it should be pointed out that the "less" we attempt to do "more" with would be more than enough in any other country.

LESS IS MORE

I lost myself in the very properties of their minds: for the moment at least I actually became them, whoever they should be, so that when I detached myself from them at the end of a half hour of intense concentration over some illness which was affecting them, it was as though I was reawakening from a sleep. For the moment I myself did not exist; nothing of myself affected me. As a consequence I came back to myself, as from any other sleep, rested.
— William Carlos Williams

How do physicians maintain their bearings in the flux of technology, economics, and regulation that distort clinical judgment? First, it is important to state what perhaps should be axiomatic: medical care is administered by human beings in the context of interpersonal relationships. William Carlos Williams, poet and physician, made no distinction between his clinical and poetic fascination with human experience. He asks himself in his autobiography: "Was I not interested in man? There the thing was, right in front of me. I could touch it, taste it, smell it. It was myself, naked, just as it was, without a lie telling itself to me in its own terms."[4] Williams identified with his patients, and if he might then be attracted or repelled, the professional attitude that every physician must call on would steady him and dictate the terms on which he could proceed. The interplay between professionalism and humanism, in a more modern context of competencies and systems, is as crucial to current medical practice as it was to Dr. Williams.

REFLECTIVE PRACTICE AND MINDFULNESS

Amidst the clamor and urgency of a busy medical practice, some physicians manage to be not only calm but also efficient. Self-awareness can bring clarity and insight to the ordinary everyday tasks that might otherwise distract and annoy.[5] Clinical medicine is an art as well as a science, and the reflective as well as effective practitioner is able to link "tacit knowledge," which comes with experience and close observation, to "explicit knowledge," which at its best is evidence-based. Evidence-based medicine, and the numbers that support its conclusions, is one of the mantras that healthcare reformers and the health insurance industry both chant. Too often physicians, young and old, miss the forest through the trees. They remain prisoners of their last case. They rely on evidence they cannot judge. However, quantified models of clinical reasoning often prove to be more distractions than guides.[6] Specious numbers provide false reassurance. To make the right medical decision at the right time, to give good advice, the physician needs to know when to steer outside the practice guidelines.

A retired and cantankerous journalist with progressive macular degeneration can no longer read. Her favorite doctor, the one she will listen to, trades books-on-tape with her. A 30-minute follow-up visit takes 10 minutes for diabetes and hypertension; 15 minutes for counseling (diet, exercise, medication), and five minutes for which books they'd like to share.

Through the development of mindfulness, of moment-to-moment nonjudgmental awareness of human experience, physicians are able to give patients the attention they deserve.

An older physician, now too often a patient himself, talked about his surgeon coming to visit, sitting down next to the bed, not standing over it, and creating the impression he had as much time as his patient needed.

Mindfulness can be taught. As Yogi Berra is reported to have said, "You can observe a lot just by noticing." Physicians can develop and nurture their capacity for mindfulness and self-awareness by practicing meditation, keeping journals, reading and sharing stories, making their own stories, shaping experience into poetry.[7] Groups such as the American Academy on Physician and Patient (AAPP) offer courses for professional development using group process and feedback, videotape review and role-play. "Mindfulness for physicians" courses, adopting the Mindfulness-Based Stress Reduction (MBSR) program developed by Jon Kabat-Zinn and Saki Santorelli at the University of Massachusetts Medical Center, are offered at the University of

Virginia School of Medicine.[8] These courses meet weekly for eight weeks and allow physicians to practice meditation and apply the lens of mindfulness to daily stress at work and home. A similar program at the University of Arizona was shown to decrease measures of psychological distress and increase empathy scores among medical students.[9]

Physicians who enroll in mindfulness courses do so out of need; they feel isolated and unsuccessful at work. Given that many doctors are perfectionists, it would be surprising if a sense of professional failure was uncommon. Given the workload, both for residents and practicing physicians, it would also be surprising if doctors did not feel at times overwhelmed by the number and complexity of the problems they are asked to solve. The opposite of mindfulness is mindlessness, the last resort of the exhausted physician. Is it really necessary for the physician to read everything he or she must sign? Obstacles to mindfulness include lack of curiosity, dogmatism, lack of imagination, and burnout with attendant anger and frustration. Mindfulness won't change the long hours doctors must keep or the demands of the profession, but it can change the set of impossible expectations that guarantee failure.

THE HEALER'S ART

To a large extent residents and medical students learn by doing. While they learn quickly from mistakes, they may also not get over their mistakes. Rachel Nemen, recognizing the vulnerability of medical students and their needs as initiates into a community of service, developed "The Healer's Art" course at the University of California, San Francisco, 12 years ago.[10] Currently 35 schools of medicine in the United States offer "The Healer's Art." This curriculum creates an opportunity for students to recognize and enhance the human dimensions of healthcare, enables professionals to explore the core values that sustain a medical career, allows students the initial experience of joining a community of service, and introduces some of the self-preservation skills that sustain reflective practice.

The University of Virginia School of Medicine recently offered "The Healer's Art" course in five evening sessions, including large and small group meetings, with volunteer faculty as mentors and discussion leaders. Poetry, drawing, reflective writing, and small group sharing were used to explore the issues involved in entering a service profession, exploring personal grief and loss, and discovering the means to nurture humanitarian and service ideals during residency training. Sixty students from the first and second year classes gave up five evenings for a course offering no academic credit. Their participation was enthusiastic, and the evaluations were glowing. The course will be offered again, to faculty as well as students. By definition, it is not and should not be a required course. It helps those who want to be helped. "The Healer's Art" may be preaching to the choir, but it also reaches the congregation. It remains to be seen if a valuable classroom experience like "The Healer's Art" will prevent battle fatigue in the clinical year.

ILLNESS NARRATIVE

Mindful practice and "The Healer's Art" emphasize self-awareness and also create opportunities to listen to the stories patients need to share. Physicians may know it is time to listen, but it is also time to see the next patient. Not only do physicians often feel tardy, they also often feel claustrophobic. The moment for listening is cluttered with clinical and administrative problems.

Mindfulness offers a means of creating the sense of space necessary to let stories unfold.[11]

A patient is ready, almost, to be discharged from the hospital to a nursing home. If only the GI bleeding would stop. The doctor is anxious to claim the nursing home bed while it is still open. The family needs a little more time, and a little more family, to decide what is best near the end of life. The physician's awareness, which she terms mindfulness, preserved the calm and caring atmosphere that allowed end-of-life questions to be raised and answered. It did mean an extra day in the hospital and a delay in the complicated transfer to the nursing home. It turned out to be necessary for both ends of the transfer to accommodate the family. The organizational ethic and the doctor-patient ethic were able to mesh. It helped that the physician requesting the delayed transfer to the nursing home was also the medical director of the nursing home.

There is a rich literature on narrative medicine, and patient stories, whether embellished for literary purpose[12] or stripped for clinical discourse (Mr. Smith is a 68-year-old White male admitted for chest pain), allow physicians to understand the illness that follows the disease.[13] In reviewing a hospital chart or a series of progress notes in clinic, the clinical story is often told without mention of work, education, interests, family — the details that add drama and meaning. Even if clinical distance is important (not every patient can be a friend), it is still important to know how an illness affects a life, what gets left behind as medical morbidity takes over. The patient's story and often the language used to tell the story, the barren woman who asks to be referred to the infidelity clinic, allow physicians to understand suffering and pay attention to recovery.

HOME VISITS

There is no better way to get patients' stories than to visit them at home.[14] But who does home visits any more? An hour and a half for a home visit means six or more patients in the office, where physicians need to be, seeing however many patients it takes to pay the rent and staff. A few doctors, by choice, convenience, organizational lapse, or generosity, manage to see patients at their homes. The Gold Foundation will pay medical schools to develop a home visit experience for residents, and grants from this foundation allow University of Virginia pediatric and internal medicine residents to leave clinic and make visits to patients at their homes. Part of the home visit grant pays for lunch. The residents see patients at home and see an attending outside the hospital, two kinds of eye-opening experiences.

PALLIATIVE CARE

At the end of life, patients not only need care at home but also well-organized and experienced hospice care. This subject was discussed previously as an example of "more with less" healthcare. Palliative care is worth mentioning twice, or three times, in an essay that explores the boundaries of professionalism and humanism. When physicians have an opportunity to take care of dying patients in their homes, meet the family, see the bedroom, walk through the kitchen, notice the dog while carefully avoiding the dog, and picture the life before its final illness, the values of the profession speak eloquently for themselves. When the physician takes a resident or medical student along, the home visit does its own teaching.

ROUND PEGS IN SQUARE HOLES

In a busy out-patient practice it is hard to look past the next patient. The doctor takes them one at a time, tries to stay on schedule, and tries to be fair to each in sequence, even though the logic of such fairness is ultimately self-defeating. If physicians aren't robbing Peter to pay Paul today, the current generation of graying boomers with high expectations and accommodating personal physicians is not apt to leave much for their children. Even if physicians and regional healthcare organizations agree on common goals and values, the marketplace pits one organization against another. Hilary Clinton called this managed competition. For whatever political and philosophical reasons, the federal government is not willing or able to develop a national health policy.

For years now there has been a growing healthcare crisis. Even though the health economy pie is getting bigger, the line for slices is longer, and, for most consumers, the slice is thinner. Meanwhile, doctors go to work, see a lot of patients, still get paid well, and there are more young, smart, idealistic applicants to medical schools than there are places. However, there are not as many applicants as there once were. The physicians of the future are at high risk to be unhappy during residency and perhaps afterward.[15] Hamsters run inside the wheel to get fed, but at least the food comes quickly. Among other learning goals, medical students must learn to be masters of delayed gratification. They graduate with six-figure debt, become indentured servants for three to 10 years, then rush off to pursue the American dream. Their training programs must persuade the ACGME that all graduates can solve the riddle of the systems-based practice competency. Regardless of systems-based competency curricula, once they leave residency, physicians survive by adapting to whichever bureaucratic matrix confronts them in practice. They join a team and figure out the incentives and disincentives that third, fourth, and fifth parties put between them and their patients. Moreover, these graduates, under oath, must promise to be good scouts. And they are, most of them, most of the time, but not without complaining.

Talking to residents about the intangible rewards of medical practice is like talking to galley slaves about the nice view of the ocean. Students arrive on the wards and quickly identify with their closest peers, the house staff, not the attending staff, and for good reason. The resident will teach them what they need to know to survive a busy night. The attending physicians get to go home at night. There, after dinner, they write chapters, think about the intangible rewards of medical practice, and perhaps share a story with husband or wife about the grateful patient they saw that day and what that felt like.

Inui talks about the hidden curriculum of medical education.[16] Students in the clinical year absorb what they need to know to get the hospital admissions tucked in for the night. They notice what the house staff and attendings do, listen to what they say, and mark the discrepancies. They learn it is OK to be cynical. In current usage, a cynic believes that human acts are selfish, survival supersedes selflessness. However, the first cynics were fourth-century Greek philosophers who believed that the essence of virtue is self-control. The first two years of medical school are lessons in Greek cynicism. Survival requires the denial of impulse. It is always time to study. Whatever pole of cynicism is handy, the students will hang on. They survive. They adapt.

The round peg will feel uncomfortable in the square hole unless it adapts quickly. Medical students learn to be average students in their first two years, and to be sleep deprived in the third; residents learn to elicit "no code" decisions immediately after introducing themselves to new patients; practicing physicians learn the hard way to code for service rendered and document the level of service.

Professionals are good enough at what they do to get paid for it. The medical profession wants to get paid, but it also expects its members to be selfless, to put the patient first (see table 8.1). The health system wants to maintain access to high quality care and also maintain its bottom line. Doctors are often stuck, or lost, between the business of medicine and the foggy idealism they brought with them as medical students. To further complicate the maze of healthcare, at each turn physicians are apt to bump into one of the 40 million uninsured Americans.

Round pegs don't fit into square holes. They get hammered. That is a difficult image near the end of a chapter. Instead, be mindful, picture this: two physicians share a small office, it's the end of the day, no charts are waiting on either desk, before they leave one of them remembers to water the bedraggled philodendron a patient gave the other years ago. Not only do they deserve a nicer plant, the plant deserves a nicer pot. One of these days. . . .

But change is difficult. It takes an internal medicine house staff program three years to change, one residency lifetime. If the new interns face what the graduating seniors faced, that seems fair, or at least arguably fair. For physicians in practice, the memories are longer and the stakes seem higher. Nostalgia is not just for the good old days with the doctor and the patient and no third parties, but also the good old days of no-questions-asked billing, more than enough hospitals and beds, and perhaps a deeper faith in the biomedical revolution. Doctors are like everyone, they resist change when change means loss of authority. When changing light bulbs they remember the old, clear, simple light. Although the profession is no longer sovereign,[17] it is still far from democratic. Medicine is not just a commodity, and patients are not just consumers. Nevertheless, healthcare is big business, at 18 percent of the GNP the biggest business in the United States. When the University of Virginia School of Medicine looks for help preparing its next generation of leaders, it asks the business school faculty. They teach round pegs to find round holes and square pegs to find square holes. More important, every peg must know what it is getting into and why it is there in the first place. To whatever extent the healthcare puzzle can be solved at the front lines, systems-based practice, mindfulness, humanism, and professionalism are the means to the solutions.

NOTES

1. T. Inui, *A Flag in the Wind: Educating for Professionalism in Medicine* (Washington, D.C.: Association of American Medical Colleges, 2003).

2. E. Spencer and R. Bigoney, "Toward a New Concept of Professionalism: Being a Physician in Today's Healthcare System," *Organizational Ethics: Healthcare, Business, and Policy* 2, no. 1 (Spring 2005): 19-29.

3. R. Lebow, *Health Care Meltdown: Confronting the Myths and Fixing Our Failing System* (Chambersburg, Pa.: Alan C. Hood, 2004).

4. W.C. Williams, *The Autobiography of William Carlos Williams* (New York: New Direction Books, 1967).

5. R. Epstein, "Mindful Practice," *Journal of the American Medical Association* 282 (1999): 833-9.

6. A. Feinstein, "Clinical Judgment Revisited: The Distraction of Quantitative Models," *Annals of Internal Medicine* 120 (1994): 799-805.

7. J. Connelly, "Being in the Present Moment: Developing the Capacity for Mindfulness in Medicine," *Academic Medicine* 74(1999): 420-4.

8. J. Kabat-Zinn, *Wherever You Go, There You Are: Mindfulness Meditation in Everyday Life* (New York: Hyperion, 1994).

9. S. Shapiro, G. Schwartz, and G. Bonne, "Effects of Mindfulness-Based Stress Reduction on Medical and Premedical Students," *Journal of Behavioral Medicine* 21, no. 6 (1998): 581-99.

10. R. Remen, "Recapturing the Soul of Medicine: Physicians Need to Reclaim Meaning in their Working Lives," *Western Journal of Medicine* 174 (2001): 4-5.

11. J. Connelly, "Narrative Possibilities: Using Mindfulness in Clinical Practice," *Perspectives in Biology and Medicine* 48 (2005): 84-9.

12. W.C. Williams, *The Doctor Stories* (New York: New Directions Books, 1984).

13. A. Kleinman, *The Illness Narratives: Suffering, Healing, and the Human Condition* (New York: Basic Books, 1999); H. Brody, "My Story is Broken, Can You Help Me Fix It? Medical Ethics and the Joint Construction of Narrative," *Literature and Medicine* 13 (1994): 220-3; R. Charon, "Narrative Medicine: Form, Function, and Ethics," *Annals of Internal Medicine* 134 (2001): 83-8; A. Verghese, "The Physician Storyteller," *Annals of Internal Medicine* 135 (2001): 1012-6.

14. D. Becker, "Home Visit," *Journal of the American Medical Association* 282 (1999): 217.

15. J. Coulehan and P. Williams, "Vanquishing Virtue: The Impact of Medical Education," *Academic Medicine* 76 (2001): 598-605.

16. See note 1 above.

17. P. Starr, *The Social Transformation of American Medicine* (New York: Basic Books, 1982).

The Patient's Perspective

9

Through the Looking Glass: The Patient's Point of View

Daniel M. Becker

A previous chapter in this book examined the ways humanism buffers professionalism amidst the melee of contemporary healthcare in the United States. The authors presented themselves as straw dogs (a cheap literary device), exemplars of primary care, devoted to their patients, but also hoping to secure some personal happiness along the way. Perhaps some material happiness too. As practitioners they'd have good days and bad days, easy cases and not so easy, people sad and happy, young and old, and old before their time.

A 60-year-old woman has been seeing one of these doctors for 20 years.[1] Last week she was admitted for an upper GI bleed. Silent reflux led to erosive esophagitis. The hospital told her to call her primary care physician for follow-up. She called the clinic and got lost in the voice mail. She called again on the appointment line and was put on hold then got disconnected. She called again on the prescription line and left a message. The nurse called her back in an hour and left a message instructing her to use the nurse appointment line, not the prescription line or the front desk appointment line. The patient called the nurse line and actually talked to the nurse, who said she had to talk to the doctor and would call her back. The nurse talked to the doctor, who looked at his schedule and said the patient would have to call first thing in the morning for a triage visit. The next morning the patient called at 0800 as instructed and talked to the nurse, who offered a late afternoon appointment, but that's when the patient's grandson gets home from school. The nurse told the doctor who said OK, he'd see her during lunch. At his clinic they eat fast. They talk with their mouths full.

The patient was a little late and the doctor noticed. If he runs over with her, he will be late for every patient that afternoon. She doesn't mind when he fusses. That means he is paying attention. She was late because she had to circle the parking garage for 30 minutes before she found a place to park. Then they kept her downstairs at registration, wanting to know her mother's maiden name and clicking at the computer in a mean way as if it was dumb and should know everyone. When the doctor heard that he got mad at registration instead of at her. He will write a letter, make a phone call. That is another thing she likes about him, his righteousness. He asked how she felt, was she taking her meds, had she returned to work. He let her undress in private. Then he checked her blood pressure, heart, lungs, abdomen, and extremities and told her she checked out OK. She didn't need the g-y-n exam. He said he couldn't remember what happened to her husband. Her chart is 20 years thick — diabetes, hypertension, sleep apnea, aches and pains, slings and arrows. She describes herself as large and unlucky. The hall nurse documented vital signs including pain, problem list, med list, and patient education in three flow sheets in front of the chart. The Joint Commission is coming. The clinic managers have been doing in-services on chart hygiene and scheduling fire drills.

The patient lives alone. Her husband was shot dead 35 years ago. An accident. He didn't have life insurance and hadn't earned enough for his widow to get a Social Security check. She raised their two kids. She cleans rooms in a hotel, a 30-minute drive, two gallons of gas there and back. Her car gets lousy mileage. If she doesn't work she doesn't have insurance. She says her insurance is lousy, and she is right. The prescription benefits are stingy. Because she works, she can't get the full discount at the university pharmacy. She could if her kids still lived at home and didn't work. When they left home she lost her Medicaid. During the Clinton era they took away her welfare and made her work. Her doctor remembers that and her asking him if he thought it was fair or not for her to lose her benefits.

Through the Looking Glass: The Patient's Point of View

She asks what about her neck? His hand is on the doorknob; his mind is on the 12:30 patient . . . patients actually, man and wife. It's the wife's appointment but the husband takes notes. They want to discuss her good cholesterol and how to make it better. They sent him some information from the internet that seems to contradict something he said last time they came to discuss their lipids.

Whose stomach is growling?

Her neck, of course, the car accident, almost killing her, she was rear-ended driving to work. She asks if it hurts enough to be disabled. She asks if he knows a lawyer. He knows a lawyer, but she should check the yellow pages. She can read, a little. She can't run a computer. She was slow at school. If she didn't make beds she'd work fast food.

He feels sorry for her. His back is killing him. Sometimes his neck hurts when he holds the phone with his shoulder while answering e-mail when he is also dictating.

She calls back the next day because the prescription for her esophagus was too expensive. Insurance wouldn't pay. They need more information, and then they might pay, but no promises. She left a message on the prescription line. The phone nurse doing prescriptions called her back and then wrote up a telephone encounter form and put it on the doctor's shelf. Between patients he takes things off the shelf and signs them or initials them or marches them back to the nurse. Recently, he changed his signature to just his initials with a long line that implies the other letters. That way he saves a second or two each time he signs. His writing is legible. Patients can read his instructions. It takes time to be understood.

Insurance doesn't pay for the esophagus pill until the much less expensive and slightly less effective pill has failed. The doctor needs to fill out a prior approval form so that the pharmacy benefit manager for that insurance company will OK the prescription. He can't find the prior approval forms for that pharmacy benefits manager. He asks the nurse where they are. She is on the phone and he tried not to interrupt, but it takes so much effort to stand there not doing anything that it makes the nurse he is waiting for nervous. She gives him the form without breaking telephone stride. She logs 300 calls a day, about 40 an hour.

He is supposed to fill out the form (takes a minute not a second less), it gets faxed, if approved they fax back the approval form, the office calls the pharmacy, the pharmacy gets the faxed approval form faxed to them, and then calls the patient to leave a message she can come get her medicine.

However, the doctor doesn't want to fill out the form. First, he wants everyone in the office to understand this is not why he went to medical school. He says his gravestone will read "died without prior approval." The nurses watch him stress and tell him to get over it. He fills out the form and uses exclamation points and rhetorical questions to really make the case for approval, that without approval the patient will die and the pharmacy benefits company will only have itself to blame.

He forgets, for the moment, that the organizational ethic and the personal ethic are supposed to share common values. He forgets, for the moment, this is about the patient, not him. His partner, watching, asks if this might be a good time to be mindful, to let go of the anger. Or, would it be more fun to kick it around for a little while? Yes.

The patient gets the medicine. It gives her diarrhea. She repeats the phone nurse ritual, choosing line #2 for prescription questions, not line #3 for same day appointments, and the phone nurse writes it up and leaves the chart on the doctor's shelf. Plan B is back to pharmacy benefits for another esophagus pill. The doctor likes to say this feels like a game of badminton. Actually, it is like two games of badminton played at the same time. Meanwhile, there are hundreds of other patients. The literature does not agree on the proper size patient panel for a general internist full-time equivalent.[2] When they ask the doctor in a boutique practice, the answer is 500. When they ask the network or system or managed-care plan, the answer is in the thousands.

The second medicine seems to work. At least, there is no more diarrhea or bleeding. The esophagus never hurt. Her neck hurts, her back too, and she takes over-the-counters: Aleve, Advil, Motrin, Tylenol. Her doctor says the generics are just as good and cheaper. She is willing to pay for the brand names.

She wakes up one day and has trouble speaking. She has some numbness in her left arm. Then it got better. The next day she calls the office and the phone nurse sends her to the ER. The doctor reads the telephone encounter form on top of her chart on his shelf. He wonders if she is left-handed. He wonders about NSAIDs[3] and hypertension and acute renal failure and stroke and heart attack. He wonders what he could have done or should have done. When he sees her at the hospital that evening after clinic, she has been wondering about disability.

Lying around all day in the hospital is a good time to wonder about retrieving her lost benefits. Does she need to drop dead first? She is not the ironic type. He is relieved that her speech has returned. When the scans don't show a stroke, she is discharged. The ward team wanted her to start aspirin, but she refused. Someone she knows got an ulcer from aspirin. The next day she cleans 10 rooms and changes sheets on 20 beds. Her arm and shoulder hurt. The neck never stops hurting.

She returns to clinic and he tells her that if she had a stroke her chance for disability would be better. She leaves some forms from Social Security she'd like him to fill out. Also, a medical leave form that her job needs, also a medical report for an insurance policy that pays her when she is sick, and finally a mortgage deferment form (her mother's house, now hers, but really the bank's). He does not know how many hours a day she can sit or stand, whether she can carry 20 pounds 100 feet and how often, whether it is pain or fatigue or weakness or shortness of breath that limits these activities. If pain, what kind of pain — muscular-skeletal and if so where and why, neuropathic and if so where and why, other and if so where and why? He does know he only wants to complete the forms once. Together they make up the answers. He doesn't charge her for the visit. She calls the next day and says she forgot to ask about the form for a disabled parking tag. He says sure, that one is easy.

When she isn't working her back doesn't hurt. She figures her neck will always hurt. Her job offers to send her to low back school. She learns how to walk, sit, stoop instead of bend. Her knees swell from all the stooping. They move her from cleaning rooms to halls. She pushes a power waxer around the lobby. Her shoulders hurt. She can't wax. She can't scratch her own back. She is constipated from the pain meds. Physical therapy helps, but she only gets six visits per condition. Her doctor, coached by the physical therapist, renames the condition. He then appeals the denial for more therapy. He sends her to pain clinic. They think the shoulder pain is from the neck. Maybe she needs an MRI. Her chart stays on his shelf.

Her doctor orders the MRI, but the medical director of her insurance company needs more information before approving the study. For example, what did the plain films show? The plain films showed 60-year-old bones and disks, some wear and tear arthritis. Are there neurological symptoms? Only pain, no weakness. How will the MRI change management? Depends on what it shows. After scheduling the MRI they call her and leave a message: the study has been postponed pending insurance approval. Then they call her back to reschedule it for the late afternoon, but she can't do it then because of her grandson. Eventually the MRI shows 60-year-old bones and disks, some wear and tear arthritis, some moderate foraminal impingement (more on the left than right), and something funny in front of the spine, a nodule too small to characterize. Radiology suggests a PET scan. The medical director of the insurance company needs more information before approving the study. The doctor faxes the MRI report in order to justify the PET, but isn't sure the fax was sent. He is suspicious of the fax machine. Truth is, he hates the fax machine. Just because it makes a noise and lights up doesn't mean it was sent. He asks the nurse to fax it again for him. She is on the telephone and he almost doesn't interrupt. The PET scan is done a week later and shows a nodule too small to characterize. Radiology suggests a follow-up study in six months.

The disability application is rejected. The pain in the neck, back, shoulders, knees is generalized. She hurts all over. At least they don't make her push the power waxer now. She keeps asking for doctor excuses. He is surprised the excuses work. If she can't clean rooms or floors, what can she do? Bathrooms.

A year after the esophagus pill was first prescribed, her doctor renews it. Her insurance won't pay without prior approval. Nurse, pharmacy benefits, and pharmacy are linked by faxes, and each fax in turn arrives on the doctor's shelf to be initialed and then filed. The patient's chart enters volume two.

She hires a lawyer from the yellow pages. The lawyer writes the doctor and requests a report on his patient's condition. The doctor writes a note on the lawyer's letter and faxes it back with a year's worth of clinic notes. The lawyer writes back with a list of questions. What is the most proximate cause of the patient's neck pain? Does this pain make it impossible to work all of the time, some of the time, none of the time? What kind of work could she do all of the time, some of the time, none of the time? What future limitations might she anticipate all of the time, some of the time, none of the time? The doctor tells the nurse to call the patient and tell her she needs to come in and keep him company while he tries to understand and answer these questions. The nurse asks if she can use a triage slot. But the patient can't come late in the afternoon because that is when her grandson gets home. She can come at noon. Now that she has a disabled parking permit, it is easy to park.

A neurosurgeon is consulted. The nerves in the neck should be decompressed. She goes to surgery, and afterward her pain drops from a 6 to a 3 on a scale of 1 to 10. The lawyer goes to court. Her doctor and neurosurgeon testify that the pain started after the accident. They are paid for the time it takes to write the lawyer, travel to court, and testify. Her doctor donates the money to the housestaff teaching fund. He can deduct the donation from his federal income tax. The settlement pays the patient for pain and suffering and lost income, after deducting the lawyer and doctor fees and expenses.

Social Security has some concerns about her disability. They send her to one of their doctors. He does an EKG and pulmonary function tests as part of his disability assessment. He asks her to walk up and down the hall carrying 10 pounds, then 20 pounds. She is winded easily. Maybe there is an underlying cardiac condition. Perhaps she needs formal exercise testing. Her lungs work fine. The EKG shows some nonspecific changes.

She is worried about her heart. Her doctor arranges for a nuclear stress test. At a low work load a slight inferior defect was noted. Perhaps inducible ischemia, or maybe breast artifact. The cardiologist reading the study suggested clinical correlation. The bill for the stress test was denied by the insurance company. The patient brought the bill to her doctor, and he wrote a letter justifying the test based on his concerns about silent ischemia or atypical angina. Perhaps the medical director was not aware that women, especially women with diabetes, are more likely than men to have atypical presentations of coronary artery disease? Sarcasm is lost on the medical director. Insurance agrees to pay. Her doctor suggests aspirin. She agrees, with some misgivings. Someone she knows got an ulcer from aspirin. Her doctor says yes, but. . . .

She tolerates the aspirin for a month and is then admitted with an upper GI bleed. She had stopped taking the esophagus pill. Even with insurance approval, the $18.00 co-pay was too much. On aspirin she developed a duodenal ulcer. She is in the hospital for two days. She can't remember the names of any of the doctors who visited her. They woke her up and asked if it hurt. Someone said she didn't need the aspirin because she didn't really have angina, she hadn't had a stroke or mini-stroke. She wonders how he knows so much if he wasn't even there? Someone else sat down on her bed and started pressing her stomach, asking if it hurt. Of course it hurts when a large stranger presses on your stomach. Someone said the esophagus pill works just as good in the duodenum, but she will need to double her dose. Her doctor came to visit one evening and explained about the aspirin and how hard it was to balance risk and benefit. She didn't like the sound of that, but appreciated his coming to see her.

She needs a prescription for the higher dose of the esophagus pill. She calls on the prescription line because insurance approves 90 pills for 90 days but not 180 pills for 90 days. The phone nurse puts the chart and the telephone encounter form and the prior approval form on the doctor's shelf.

The second GI bleed, and the TIA,[4] and the arthritis in her spine, and the clinic progress notes that document her aches and pains and limitations, persuade Social Security. She gets her monthly check and Medicare. She quits the hotel job. With the whiplash settlement from the automobile insurance company, she pays off her mortgage. She does some private housecleaning work because she likes to stay busy; gas is expensive. During Bush and under Medicare she gets a break on her pills, not much, but it helps. Gas is more expensive.

The hospital, now renamed a health system, sends the patient a patient satisfaction survey. She wasn't sure what it was at first or what it was for. She called her doctor and left a message asking if it was OK to fill it out. His nurse called her back and said yes. Actually, he said to tell the patient to burn it. She answers truthfully. He is hard to reach on the telephone some of the time but not all of the time. It is hard to get an appointment with him most of the time. He is always in a rush. The nurses are nice all the time. She would say he is above average. She would say her previous doctor was below average because he never saw her. After filling out the questionnaire she threw it away. She hates forms. Besides, it's none of the hospital's business and what the heck is a health system anyway.

Her chart failed a health system audit. Her doctor failed to meet documentation guidelines for complete review of systems and family history. Medicare sent her a letter suggesting she was over-billed by her doctor. She read the first paragraph and threw it away. She gets more mail than she can read from those people.

NOTES

1. The patient discussed in this chapter is a composite of numerous patients and their clinical and administrative dilemmas.
2. R. Snyderman, G.F. Sheldon, and T.A. Bischoff, "Gauging Supply and Demand: The Challenging Quest to Predict the Future Physician Workforce," *Health Affairs* 21 (2002): 167-168.
3. Non-steroidal anti-inflammatory drugs.
4. Transient ischemic attacks.

Residency Training and Outcomes Assessment

10

Educating for Systems-Informed Professionalism

Donna T. Chen and Ann E. Mills

The ACGME competency on systems-based practice requires that residents learn "how to partner with . . . managers and . . . providers to assess, coordinate, and improve health care."[1] Since healthcare and its outcomes depend on systems to deliver it, this requirement in effect acknowledges that future physicians ought to work to improve the systems surrounding care with the goal of delivering optimal care. Because "optimal care" implies that patients receive care in the right amounts at the right time, "optimal care" is cost-effective *quality* care. Because *quality* care in the healthcare context cannot be divorced from medical professionalism, any "improvement" having to do with the systems that surround healthcare and its delivery must take into account medical professionalism and the values associated with it.

In chapter two, "Towards Systems-Informed Professionalism," Donna Chen, Ann Mills, and Patricia Werhane developed a framework that can be used to help residents and other physicians as they try to improve these systems (see figure 10.1, below).[2] This framework, which we call "systems-informed professionalism," has two components. The first component includes the framework we have borrowed from Robert Kaplan and David Norton, which identifies the elements needing attention for suc-

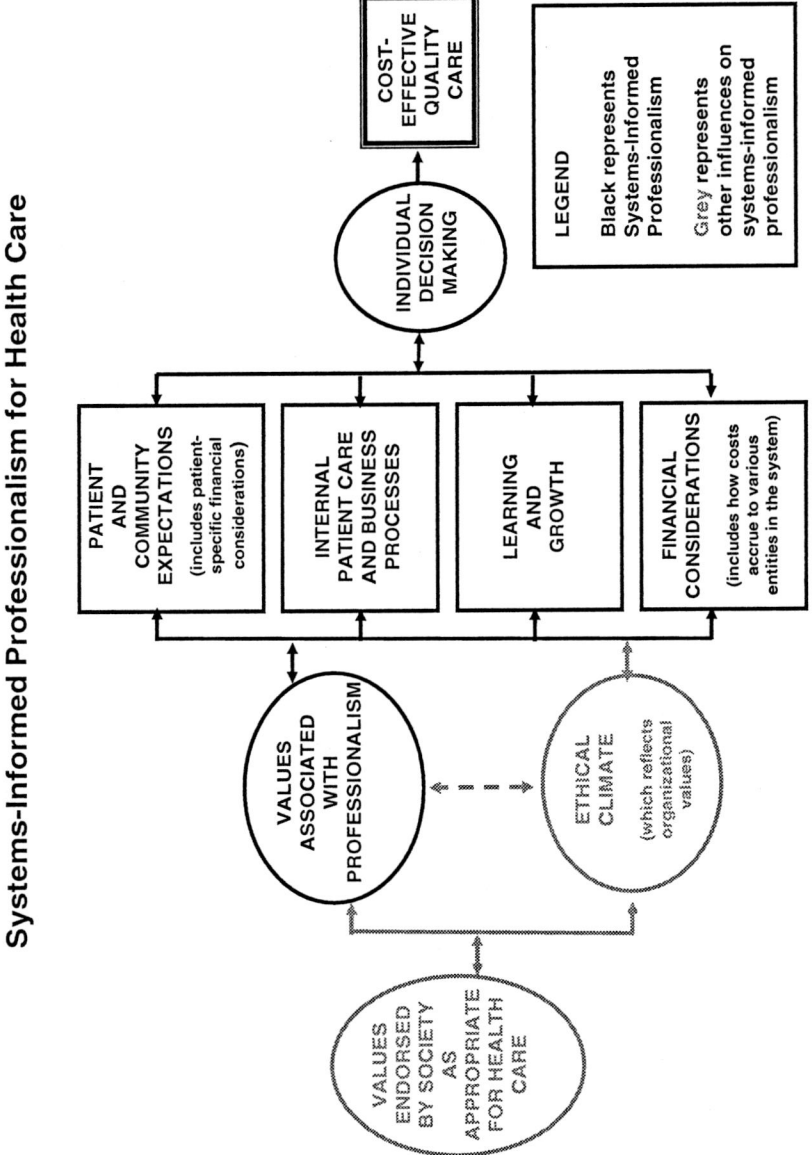

Figure 10.1

cessful functioning of an organizational system.[3] But, as described in chapter two, these elements can be directly tied to any human system — at whatever level is under discussion. These four components are:

- The purpose of the system, or, in this context, the desired or envisioned goals and outcomes associated with the patient or community;
- The way in which the system achieves its purpose, or, in this context, the internal patient care and business practices;
- The special needs of humans, or, in this context, the special needs (learning and growth) that individuals working in healthcare, including physicians, must acquire to help achieve the purpose of the system; and, finally,
- The minimum survival needs, or, in this context, the financial needs of the healthcare organization.

The second component of systems-informed professionalism for physicians *is* professionalism, which includes the values associated with it. These values, as outlined by the ACGME, now reflect both traditional professional values and attention to the ethical principles that are associated with business practices.[4] However, if we want residents and other physicians to develop a perspective that is characterized by systems-informed professionalism, how do we help them develop it? What other knowledge, skills, and sensitivities must residents have in order to use this perspective? What is it that we want residents to know and do? This chapter addresses these issues.

We divide this chapter into four sections. In this first section we describe the knowledge, skills, and sensitivities physicians need in order to be able to use the framework and acquire the perspective provided by systems-informed professionalism. In the next section, we use the Dreyfus model of skills acquisition to outline how we think this perspective can be integrated into the medical education and training process. In this section we outline the knowledge, skills, and sensitivities for developing this perspective that we consider appropriate at each step in acquiring this perspective. The third section discusses the mechanisms available to embed these ideas into residency training. The fourth section of this essay describes what we consider to be important benefits for the resident from adopting this perspective. We will conclude, however, with the familiar theme, that the acquisition of this perspective will only go so far in helping residents and other physicians confront the challenges of delivering cost-effective quality care in the context of systems-based practice.

WHAT IS REQUIRED TO USE A PERSPECTIVE CHARACTERIZED BY "SYSTEMS-INFORMED PROFESSIONALISM"

Systems-informed professionalism provides a framework for a perspective that we believe is necessary for the physician to conceptualize professionalism in today's complex healthcare world. It provides a way to conceptualize what and how values and system components influence, facilitate, or limit a physician's decision making. However, as mentioned before in chapter two, a framework is just that, a framework. It does not ensure that appropriate values are represented, that correct system components are included in an analysis of a systems problem, or that suitable decisions are made. Many other skills, sensitivities, and pieces of knowledge are needed. For residency training, these other knowledge, skills, and sensitivities are embodied within the other ACGME competencies.

In particular, for systems-informed professionalism to be useful, the resident will have to learn the skills and sensitivities needed to make moral decisions and to practice medicine with professionalism. These requirements do not change. They are only made more complex by the fact that medicine is currently practiced within a systems context. For example, residents still must learn the clinical practice of medicine that is informed by the values and commitments associated with professionalism. Systems-informed professionalism helps a resident understand and react to these complex requirements by providing a framework that captures the elements of a system and their interactions. Moreover, if the values associated with professionalism are incorporated, it provides the resident with criteria for making and evaluating decisions.

The need to work to improve healthcare systems represents a new commitment for residents, and, indeed, all physicians. Up until recently, physicians did not view themselves as being responsible for the healthcare delivery system, or even necessarily for the organizations in which they practice medicine. There are, of course, complex questions concerning whether this ought to be part of a physician's responsibility. However, as Thomas Inui notes in his monograph, *A Flag in the Wind: Educating for Professionalism in Medicine,*[5] regardless of what personal intentions physicians may have, they "will be judged — in some important measure — by the qualities of the organization in which [they] work."[6] Inui concludes that organizational change founded on professional values is required, and that physicians ought to play a role.

Similarly, whether intentionally or not, the ACGME addresses the question of responsibility through its requirement that residents work to improve care. However, if care is delivered through systems, improving care will sometimes mean improving systems. We are not suggesting that residents, or even physicians, for that matter, always can or should assume responsibility for the excellent functioning of the systems that surround them. But at the least, residents must be able to understand how the systems facilitate or limit their ability to provide quality care. They must be able to acknowledge that a desired clinical outcome can be jeopardized or supported by the systems that surround the physician-patient encounter, and learn to understand how. If residents cannot make this link between the systems that surround them and their actions and decision making, then they will be unsuccessful in acquiring a perspective necessary for practicing medicine that is consistent with professional values in a systems context. Furthermore, because we agree that physicians ought to take some responsibility for healthcare systems and, at the least, to take initial steps to helping to improve these systems — for example, by reporting when they feel that the system is limiting their ability to provide quality care consistent with their professional values — we agree that residents ought to learn what it takes to help improve systems.

Systems-informed professionalism provides a framework for this requirement — the requirement of improving the systems of care. However, the ability to participate in, negotiate, or initiate a change in healthcare systems requires other knowledge, skills, and sensitivities, some of which we believe make sense to incorporate into undergraduate and graduate medical education, and others that we believe can be left for advanced training and other life-long learning mechanisms.

For example, moral reasoning skills are crucial for physicians in their practice of medicine and should be learned as part of their professional development. Similar skills are also required when working to improve healthcare systems. David Ozar, in his chapter, "The Challenges of a Residency Education Program for Competencies in Organizational Ethics," discusses a curricular approach to developing knowledge, skills, and sensitivities required by moral reasoning in the context of organizational practice. Systems-informed professionalism assumes that these skills and sensitivities are possessed by physicians and are being learned by residents. For example, using systems-informed professionalism in everyday clinical decision making or in systems improvement requires the ability to "stand back," to "disengage," to view the system and its interactions dispassionately. It also requires what Werhane calls *moral imagination,* "the ability in particular circumstances to discover and evaluate possibilities not merely determined by that circumstance, or limited by its operative mental models, or merely framed by a set of rules or rule-governed concerns."[7]

Moral imagination entails a three-stage process. First, moral imagination can be initiated by recognizing that an experience, situation, or event presents some kind of moral problem or dilemma. Second, moral imagination is, by and large, a process that facilitates moral reasoning by helping us out of a particular framing box, leading us to refocus our attention, critique, revise, and reconstruct other operative mental models. These activities lead to the third stage, the development of more creative normative perspectives.[8]

Moral imagination, however, is not merely "second guessing." It also should entail work at developing fresh solutions based on revised or even different mind sets. To be morally imaginative involves evaluating new possibilities or solutions from a normative perspective, judging not only the possibilities, but also the way in which they are framed and the kinds of outcomes they are likely to produce.[9]

In the third stage, one begins to critique the situation, its dominant mental models, and the alternatives that present themselves. During this process, one begins to step out of the situation and its scripts ("scripts" refer to the anticipation of how a situation will evolve), working toward a solution that was not evident when the process began, often a solution that involves another mental model or worldview heretofore only latently available in the situation and context.[10]

Thus, moral imagination requires the ability to disengage from the context in which one finds oneself — to step back from a particular situation and take on another perspective, or, at least, to begin a critical evaluation of the situation and its operative mind sets. However, as Werhane points out, no one individual, no company or government or nation, can ever disengage completely from an event or conflict or dilemma. Our revisions, critiques, and evaluations are still context-driven by historical circumstances, culture, surrounding political and social pressures, and values perspectives. Nevertheless, investigating, analyzing, and coming to some sort of resolution concerning a problem, conflict, or dilemma requires the individual to attempt disengagement from it.

Systems-informed professionalism can help with the activities required by moral imagination in the healthcare context by providing a framework that can anchor the process of disengaging and guide the process of reasoning. Because of the complexity of the healthcare system, having a framework that incorporates both values and system structures can provide the resident with a platform to step back upon, so that, in practice, "disengagement" does not mean giving up. It can facilitate the "seeing" of the connections that must be made before solutions or alternatives are glimpsed. It can provide a framework upon which to build an alternative mental model that might guide decision making, and, because professionalism is involved, it offers evaluative criteria.

In chapter eight, "Professionalism, Humanism, Mindfulness, and the Healthcare Melee," Daniel Becker and Matthew Goodman discuss concepts they call "mindfulness" and "reflective practice." Developing this skill, being mindful, without prejudgment or prejudice, allows physicians to step back from a situation and reflect. Mindfulness sets the stage for disengagement and allows residents to put a space between themselves and the event at hand. This space may allow residents to think critically and dispassionately, so that they are able use moral imagination. Systems-informed professionalism supports its use in the service of an appropriate analysis and resolution of a systems-based problem.

SYSTEMS-INFORMED PROFESSIONALISM AND THE DREYFUS MODEL

This section of the chapter answers the question of what we believe physicians ought to know about the systems-informed professionalism framework and how we anticipate they will learn to use it. To help us, we use the Dreyfus model of skills acquisition. The Dreyfus model outlines the developmental stages of learning involved in acquiring knowledge and skills, and has been employed to characterize physician development[11] and the development of moral maturity and ethical expertise.[12] The stages in the Dreyfus model are:

- novice,
- advanced beginner,
- competent,
- proficient,
- expert.

The Dreyfus model, as applied to physicians' development, generally associates medical students with the beginner and advanced beginner stages. Residents are expected to reach the competent level by the end of their residency. Life-long learning brings physicians to the proficient and expert levels, as needed.

Obviously, when new ideas, concepts, knowledge, or skills are added to the repertoire of physicians' competencies, the stages of learning will not map neatly onto these levels of the educational process, particularly for physicians who are beyond the early stages. This means that residents may start a training program with varying levels of prior knowledge and skills in certain areas, and may not have reached the stage of advanced beginner, particularly when new concepts are continually introduced into the medical education process. These considerations will always complicate residency training, particularly in light of the ACGME goals of attaining certain levels of educational outcomes by the end of residency training. Nevertheless, the developmental process of learning will likely follow the same trajectory.

As described above, systems-informed professionalism requires incorporating many of the other competencies needed by physicians in today's healthcare world. Below, we suggest how these competencies and the perspective offered by system-informed professionalism can be acquired. We illustrate with a case.

A patient is unexpectedly ready to be discharged from the hospital on Saturday. However, the patient can only be discharged if the intravenous heparin can be converted to low-molecular-weight heparin until the warfarin level is therapeutic. Low-molecular-weight heparin may not be covered by insurance, and, when covered, it frequently requires pre-approval from the insurance company. No one from the insurance company is available over the weekend to provide such approval.

NOVICE

Medical students more or less enter medical school as novices. In describing this stage as related to clinical care, Paul Batalden and colleagues[13] note, "in the novice stage, the freshman medical student begins to learn the process of taking a history and memorizes the elements, chief complaint, history of present illness, review of systems, and family and social history."[14] In other words, they learn the components of gathering a medical history that later informs clinical decision making.

For systems-informed professionalism, medical students learn the components of systems-based practice and professionalism. They learn abstractly what various groups and individuals have said about professionalism. They learn about systems, their purposes, their elements and how they interact, and what they need to survive. They learn about the macro system and they learn about micro systems, and they learn about how the interactions of both may affect clinical care. They learn that entities and individuals, other than themselves and their patients, may affect clinical care decisions. The medical student learns abstractly that a tension exists between cost and quality in the delivery of care, and, in the context of systems-informed professionalism, medical students learn, in the abstract, how this tension affects their decision making, and how the values of professionalism can be helpful in analyzing the conflicts inherent in this tension.

The process of learning about systems-informed professionalism occurs parallel to the process of learning about moral reasoning and moral decision making, and the roles of moral imagination and reflective practice. This means that medical students must also be learning to recognize the moral dimensions of clinical, administrative, and other systems-based situations in which they will find themselves.

Medical students, when presented with the above case, should be able to understand that appropriate care involves interactions and decisions among a group of entities — that appropriate care does not depend on the physician alone, and that clinical care may be compromised as a result. They should be able to recognize the operational (we use the term "operational" to refer to how the elements of a system(s) interact in a given situation) and moral dimensions of the situation, and the differences between the two. They should be able to identify the values in conflict and the sources of the values. Further, they should begin to be able to identify when problems represent isolated events or systems problems. Finally, they should begin to identify the types of decisions and actions, both individual and systems-based, that would be required to act in accordance with values associated with medical professionalism.

For example, in this case, the medical student should begin to recognize that both operational conflicts and values conflicts contribute to the difficulties. The operational level conflicts are readily apparent: Saturday discharge is precluded by a financing system that provides selective coverage for treatment options and requires pre-approval for certain treatments, yet it is not available at certain times for necessary communication. The values conflicts are also readily apparent, although somewhat more complex and diverse. For example, earlier discharge from the hospital, when medically allowable, is consistent with the values of stakeholders on many levels. Generally, it is consistent with the patient's values of not staying in the hospital unnecessarily. It is consistent with good clinical care, as earlier discharge lessens the risk of nosocomial infection. It is consistent with the hospital and community values of having a hospital bed available, or at least not occupied unnecessarily. In this case, the physician's professional values would also be fulfilled by early discharge — it provides clinically appropriate care that is consistent with patients' values, it opens up a hospital bed, and it is more cost-effective (low-molecular-weight heparin is less expensive than hospitalization to allow for intravenous heparin). The values conflict derives from the interactions with a financing system that does not seem to be operating with values that are consistent with providing quality cost-effective care.

Does this case represent a "systems problem"? A systems problem is one that is likely to occur again and again without some kind of intervention. In this situation, one can well imagine that the case or a similar case will occur next week without intervention. Since this problem is likely to reoccur, it is not an isolated event, it is a systems problem.

The medical student should also be able to identify the options available and their consequences. For example, in this case, options range from working within the system, including (1) keep

Educating for Systems-Informed Professionalism

the patient in the hospital until Monday, when the conversation with the appropriate insurance company personnel can occur, or (2) send the patient home with the low-molecular-weight heparin, risking the possibility that the insurance company does not cover this treatment, or will not cover it in this situation, since there was no pre-approval. Even if the physician agrees to contact the insurance company post-hoc and advocate for the patient in the case of option (2), there is no guarantee that the patient will not get stuck with the bill. And, conceivably, in the case of option (1), the hospital may not get paid for the "extra" medically unnecessary hospital days, although the need for intravenous medication would generally qualify as medically indicated inpatient treatment. However, in this situation, the "need" for intravenous medication is purely operationally derived. Both of these options are suboptimal.

The novice knows that neither solution addresses the systemic problem. And, although the novice might be able to glimpse a systems solution, the novice is not yet in a position to fully develop and reason it through. The novice is not yet in a position to anticipate the consequences of a solution on all the elements of a system nor their interactions. To summarize, the novice must be:

1. Learning the values associated with medical professionalism,
2. Learning the entities that make up the delivery system,
3. Able to identify the elements of a system and how these elements might interact,
4. Learning how to identify when outcomes are compromised, as well as when professionalism might be threatened, and begin to be able to identify the operational and moral dimensions of the problem,
5. Learning and identifying the values in conflict and the sources of those values,
6. Able to distinguish between a systems problem and an isolated event,
7. Able to identify the available range of decisions and actions, and
8. Able to evaluate whether the available choices are consonant with the values associated with medical professionalism.

ADVANCED BEGINNER

The advanced beginner stage correlates with the years of clinical clerkships, when medical students learn by doing. According to Batalden and colleagues, "in the advanced beginner stage, the ... student begins to see aspects of common situations, such as those facing hospitalized patients (admissions, rounds, discharge) that cannot be defined objectively apart from concrete situations and can only be learned through experience. Maxims emerge from that experience to guide the learner."[15]

To move beyond novice to advanced beginner, the medical student must be familiar with the goals of the systems surrounding the delivery of care. The advanced beginner must also be able to identify the values associated with these goals — and how they reflect medical professionalism or not. Knowing the goals of the system helps the future physician identify when these goals are not reached. Knowing the values of the system helps the future physician identify when his or her professionalism might be compromised.

But the advanced beginner takes several more steps. As medical students begin to learn the clinical practice of medicine by working with patients, they begin to experience the effects of the systems that surround them and the conflicts in operations and in values that occur in systems-based practice. They begin to experience problems and conflicts as they try to deliver good outcomes. They are beginning to be engaged by patients and their outcomes as well as the systems that surround them.

Important educational outcomes of the advanced beginner medical student stage in general are to begin to apply the abstract concepts and knowledge they have learned to date in specific situations. And they begin to recognize the common patterns and deviations from these patterns — the common presentation of the common case, the uncommon presentation of the common case, and the common presentation of the uncommon case. No one expects medical students to have more than a passing familiarity with the uncommon presentation of the uncommon case.

Similarly, recognition of patterns and deviations should occur with regard to systems-informed professionalism. For example, medical students should learn how to identify when optimal outcomes have and have not been achieved in cases with which they are involved. In addition to recognizing when optimal outcomes have or have not been achieved, medical students in the advanced beginner stage should begin to understand what worked on a systems-level to allow achievement of an optimal outcome, and what failed to work when optimal outcomes have not been achieved. The systems-informed professionalism framework can provide a structure for these types of analyses. For example, when optimal outcomes have been achieved, one can use the systems-informed professionalism framework to elucidate how values associated with medical professionalism have been reflected in the four areas of the system, how the values associated with professionalism are reflected in the ethical climate, and how these interactions combine to allow for individual decision making that leads to cost-effective quality care.

For example, in the above case, the goal of the organizational system, as well as the physician, should be quality cost-effective care. However, it is likely that this goal will be compromised because there appear to be only two choices, and both are suboptimal. The advanced beginner knows what the choices are and that both choices are not optimal or consistent with medical professionalism. In addition, the advanced beginner also knows that this appears to be a systems problem. The advanced beginner begins to understand the consequences of a systems problem and what might be involved to solve it, and how interactions among the various elements of the system will be affected. The advanced beginner begins to use the framework supplied by systems-informed professionalism to begin the process of moral reasoning.

But, to do so, the advanced beginner also begins to step back enough from a non-optimal situation to be able to identify the operational and values conflicts embedded within the situation. The engaged advanced beginner who has experience with patients, who has accepted that systems surround their encounters with patients, must learn to be able to disengage. Unlike novices, who have learned lessons in the abstract, advanced beginners are dealing with real situations, and, when faced with a case like the one above, may initially become frustrated and angry. They have been taught to seek optimal outcomes. Advanced beginners know that, in cases like the one above, an optimal outcome will not occur. Frustration and anger can lead future physicians to develop cynicism;[16] frustration and anger can also prevent the disengagement necessary for problem-solving.

On the other hand, emotions like anger and frustration can be useful. They can signal to the advanced beginner that something might be wrong. Indeed, it has been noted that one of the challenges for medical educators is to teach advanced beginner medical students to recognize anger and frustration as signals that something is not optimal, or at least not acceptable.[17]

Thus, it is here, in this stage, that the medical student also begins to learn the process of recognizing why frustration and anger are evoked by a particular case. Here the medical student becomes aware of the need for disengagement from the particulars of a situation. It is at this point that moral imagination can be triggered. It is here that "mindfulness" can help give the space to begin the moral reasoning process required by moral imagination. And, since we are dealing with a systems problem in the context of healthcare, systems-informed professionalism can give that process the necessary structure. To summarize, the advance beginner must be:

1. Familiar with the goals of a system,
2. Able to ascertain when outcomes are not consistent with the goals of the system,
3. Able to identify the values of the system,
4. Able to understand when those values are misaligned with the values associated with medical professionalism,
5. Begin to learn to disengage from the apparent problem in service of engaging moral imagination and reflective practice,[18] and, finally,
6. Able to begin to reason through systems solutions.

COMPETENT

Residency training should take physicians from advanced beginner to the stage of competency. Batalden and colleagues note, "in the competent stage, the resident physician learns to plan the approach to each patient's situation. Risks are involved, but supervisory practices are put in place to protect the patient. Because the resident has planned the care, the consequences of the plan are knowable to the resident and offer the resident a learning opportunity."[19]

The resident will have a familiarity with the values and issues associated with medical professionalism. The resident will be familiar with the general structure and processes of the healthcare delivery system and its interactions, although many will be encountering a new organizational system in the transition from medical student to resident. The resident will have learned the elements of a system and the resident will have some experience "reflecting on practice." However, it is not until residency that physicians begin to take primary responsibility for making decisions. It is this level of engagement in which residents begin to recognize values conflicts and ethical dimensions implicitly. In the competent stage, residents will begin to use systems-informed professionalism to inform their decision making, analyze a problem, and come to some sort of resolution.

As described by the Dreyfus model, residents learn to feel good when things go well, and to feel bad when things go badly.[20] These are key steps to developing skill in ethical decision making and ethical action. Feeling badly about an outcome or a process should trigger for the resident, initially with the support and assistance of the treating team and particularly the attending physician, an analysis of the situation, including the operational and ethical dimensions, using the framework supplied by systems-informed professionalism. Early on, residents will need to disengage from the emotions of the situations in order to engage moral imagination and reflective practice; with experience, they will begin to be able to engage moral imagination and reflective practice while remaining emotionally involved.

For instance, the competent resident in the case above will feel badly when the situation described arises. He or she will understand that a decision to discharge the patient has implications for the patient if the low-molecular-weight heparin is not covered, and a decision to keep the patient in the hospital has implications for the patient in basic discomfort and risk of exposure to nosocomial illness, and for the hospital and community if a needed bed is unavailable. He or she may also feel frustrated and angry that the insurance company does not seem to be reflecting values associated with medical professionalism or values endorsed by society as appropriate to healthcare.

If the situation is unfamiliar, the competent resident will pull back from the situation and will try to reason through the problem and avoid the negative consequences he or she sees as a result of any decision that is made. In this case, the resident understands that the risk of unfortunate consequences must be endured by the patient, hospital, and/or community. By thinking more about the situation, the resident might see that he or she could discharge the patient and then follow through aggressively with the insurance company; however, even then there are no guarantees. In any case, the competent resident will try to ensure that this situation becomes an isolated event by learning to anticipate these types of situations, and possibly by ordering medications that must be pre-approved on Thursday afternoon or Friday morning. Nevertheless, the resident likely understands that this is not the best solution. Such cases are frequently not predictable, and medication pre-approved on Thursday may be inappropriate by Friday evening — even though discharge is still viable. The resident understands that others will find themselves in a similar situation and continues to feel discomfort with the barriers to providing quality care that is cost-effective.

Finally, the competent resident will begin to identify aspects of systems-based practice that are best addressed on a systems level. Translating the discomfort engendered when faced with troubling situations into advocacy for the patient, which includes working within the constraints of the systems to provide for the best outcomes possible under the circumstances, *and* into advocacy for the patient and future patients by helping to effect systems-level changes, at the least by alerting those with skill and authority within a system about the systematic barriers to providing high quality cost-effective care, will allow the resident to act in ways consistent with systems-informed professionalism.

To summarize, the competent resident:

1. Begins to use systems-informed professionalism to anticipate the consequences of a decision, and
2. Begins to come to some resolution of the problem.

PROFICIENT AND EXPERT

As described by Batalden and colleagues, "in the proficient stage, the specialist physician early in practice struggles with developing routines that can streamline the approach to the patient. Managing the multiple distracting stimuli in a thoughtful way is intellectually and emotionally absorbing. . . . In the expert stage, the mid-career physician has learned to recognize patterns of discrete clues and to move quickly, using what he or she might call 'intuition' to do the work. The physician is attuned to distortions in patterns or to slow down when things 'don't fit' the expected pattern."[21]

The proficient professional will seek to understand why communication about important patient care issues is impossible over the weekend. The proficient professional will understand that, in this case, the risk of financial injury and other potential harms is borne entirely by the patient and the hospital, and so there appears to be no incentive for the insurer to arrange appropriate communication. However, using the elements of systems-informed professionalism, the proficient professional might be able to show that this is not necessarily true. For instance, the proficient professional might be able to show that it is in the interests of both the hospital and the insurer to arrange for appropriate communication. For example, the proficient professional might be able to show that, in addition to satisfying several measures of quality, providing for low-molecular-weight heparin in this situation is more cost-effective than hospitalization for intravenous heparin, and these savings would accrue to the insurance company.

The proficient professional may also see other hidden or opportunity costs as well. For instance, physicians or residents who must in these situations waste time and energy advocating for their patients incur a cost, which is borne by the hospital. The physician might equally be able to show that, in cases where medication issues were decided in advance, adverse events might occur that have the potential to increase costs to the managed-care company as well as to the patient. The physician might be able to demonstrate that little change would be required to open communication between the hospital and the insurer. For instance, it might be that pre-approval could be given by lower level personnel on Saturday and Sunday pending approval by a reviewer on Monday. In this way, weekend requests can be logged for the insurance company, the most problematic types of cases can be reviewed, and the insurance company can also assess the impact of such clinical situations from its perspective — ideally taking into account quality of care as well as costs. This might result in cost-savings to both the hospital and insurer. It could reduce the chances of adverse events. In situations when approval was forthcoming, it would free the residents and other physicians from post-hoc advocacy. It would require little change in the internal business processes of insurers; it would require no addition of special skills. And, from the patient and systems perspective, it would further the goal of quality cost-effective care.

The proficient professional is asking and answering a series of questions about the problem. And these questions correspond to how the elements of systems function together. The physician has pinpointed desirable outcomes — which, in this case, have to do with the patient and community, not the physician changing his or her behavior. The physician is asking: What changes in internal business practices or patient care procedures must occur to achieve these outcomes? Will the change require persons involved to learn special skills? and, What are the financial implications of the change? In addition, the physician is ensuring that any change reflects the values associated with medical professionalism. The proficient professional has the ability to recognize a problem in the context of systems, to step back from the problem, to use systems-informed professionalism to reason the problem through, and to evaluate a proposed solution against the values associated with professionalism. In summary, the proficient professional will use systems-informed professionalism to *respond* to what the professional considers a systemic problem. The expert will use systems-informed professionalism to *anticipate* problems in the design of systems surrounding the delivery of care. For instance, in the above case, the expert level professional would have been able to foresee that the problem would likely occur and would have sought to prevent it before it occurred.

TEACHING AND EVALUATING THE INCORPORATION OF THE SYSTEMS-INFORMED PROFESSIONALISM PERSPECTIVE DURING RESIDENCY TRAINING

The systems-informed professionalism framework can be taught using already existing mechanisms and tools. For instance, analyses of cases during morbidity and mortality conferences can be structured according to the systems-informed professionalism framework. Glick, in discussing how outcomes data should influence teaching, suggests using cases that illustrate systems failures in several care sites that involve multiple professionals.[22] Residents can address the case through questions associated with the areas we have described. Internal patient care and business processes can be analyzed to ascertain where breakdowns occur. The financial perspective can be used to assess the financial harm to the institution — and the costs of making corrections or not. And the framework can help them to imagine alternatives that explicitly address how the values associated with professionalism can be better reflected in the new system.

There are other tools that are widely prevalent in academic health centers that can be used for formative evaluation and learning. Resident educators can use continuity clinic chart self-audits and resident learning portfolios. Other tools include multidisciplinary in-patient rounds, monthly nursing evaluation of residents, and quality assessment improvement exercises.[23] These tools also can be modified to incorporate the systems-informed professionalism framework. For instance, when assessing a case, the resident could be asked what financial implications were involved, or whether or not the patient was affected by a malfunctioning process, or whether or not the patient was subject to a process that did not reflect professional values.

Multidisciplinary rounds or attending rounds can look at cases from these four perspectives as well. For instance, it would be entirely appropriate for residents to ask about the financial ramifications of a specific case or what the patient felt after a specific incident, or whether or not a specific case indicated that research had to be done on the processes of care. Nursing evaluations can demonstrate whether or not the resident is aware of processes of care and the teamwork that is necessary to make them function.

In addressing the competencies, some program directors have encouraged their residents to sit on quality committees, or to take part in systems improvement exercises.[24] A quality committee or a systems improvement exercise will raise (or *should* raise) exactly the kinds of questions associated with the system-informed professionalism perspective we are developing. For instance, any quality committee that is concerned with improvement will investigate a possible systems malfunction. It would be hoped, too, that the committee will be concerned with the impact of either the deficiency or the recommendation for improvement on the other three areas of the systems. It is less likely that these committees currently will explicitly tie their recommendations to the values associated with medical professionalism, although the values expressed should be those associated with provision of quality cost-effective care.

It very well may be that resident educators believe that specialized skill sets are needed to address the competencies — especially the systems-based practice competency. In the above example, for instance, residents who sit on quality committees will almost certainly learn about the tools associated with quality improvement. For instance, they will surely be exposed to the individual institution's "quality plan." (This is generally a repeating four-step process; gather the facts, plan the modification, implement the modification, monitor the modification. The four steps are then repeated until managers are satisfied that the system is working correctly.) They might be exposed to terms like "root cause analysis" (an attempt to capture the element or component in a system which is defective) or "quality circles" (a team, generally interdisciplinary, that is assigned to improve a system or process). They might be taught the importance of data collection in considering an improvement or new initiative. This exposure will certainly give residents the language and the skills to investigate internal practices. But our concern is that changes — both the processes associated with the change, and the outcomes expected — are explicitly linked to the values associated with medical professionalism — including the ethical principles associated with business principles. The physician should learn to always be assessing proposed changes in light of the values associated with medical professionalism.

The ACGME has emphasized outcomes as the focal point for resident evaluation and improvement, in some cases using clinical outcomes as educational outcomes. However, it is unacceptable to hold residents accountable for systems-based outcomes they cannot control. We do not dispute that evidence relating to outcomes is important in any system, including systems associated with healthcare. Bu, as Ann Mills and Mary Rorty demonstrated in their chapter, "Business Practices, Ethical Principles, and Professionalism," even if processes produce ethically acceptable outcomes, the way in which they produce them may not be ethically acceptable. This argues that processes as well as outcomes must support or reflect professional values. For instance, a plan that is designed to cut costs by bypassing what can be viewed as an unnecessary procedure can be explicitly shown to uphold or reflect these values in both process and outcome. Thus, even in this day of outcomes-based assessments, there is a role for attention to process — in this case the processes associated with clinical care and business practices, as well as the processes associated with learning and growth — educational processes.

The literature associated with teaching the system-based practice competency is relatively slim. But many innovative ideas that are being tried. For instance, Roy Ziegelstein and Nicholas Fiebach use the "village" metaphor to teach residents the systems-based practice competency. Using this metaphor reminds residents of the importance of the larger community in providing care, and so begins to address the systems-based practice

Educating for Systems-Informed Professionalism

competency,[25] and, within the framework of systems informed-professionalism, the internal patient care and business practices area. Gary Dunnington and Reed Williams present a more complete approach. In their residency program for surgeons, they have expanded their didactic curriculum to include issues of ethics and professionalism. To learn about systems-based practice, they have their residents serve on one of the hospital quality improvement/patient safety committees for a year, and, in teams of two, design a project for presentation at grand rounds that highlights a healthcare systems error and analyze its root cause.[26]

Interestingly, while each of these approaches could explicitly link the values associated with medical professionalism to systems-based practice, instead they seem to reinforce that the values associated with professionalism are different — that they are independent of systems-based practice. The result seems to be either that professionalism and the values associated with it *can* be segregated (for instance, while Dunnington and Williams have incorporated an eight-unit, case-based approach to ethics in their curriculum, they do not appear to take explicit advantage of the important lessons for professionalism in their systems-based practice curriculum, nor for the implications of the systems-based learning on core concepts of medical professionalism) or that professionalism is so embedded in what is being done that its explicit recognition is not necessary (for instance, Ziegelstein and Fiebach mention that most resident educators understand and are familiar with the competency on professionalism, yet do not appear to make explicit how the values associated with medical professionalism are reflected in their systems-based practice curriculum.)

In our opinion, both of these approaches seem incomplete — especially if physicians go on to work in systems that allow enough flexibility so that professional judgment can be exercised. Physicians must learn what it means and feels like in terms of their practice and sense of professionalism to tie systems-based practice explicitly to the values associated with medical professionalism. The only way this will happen is to insist that values associated with professionalism are explicitly taken into account and reflected in the systems that are designed to deliver healthcare, and that physicians learn to assess whether these values are reflected in their systems-based practice of medicine.

BENEFITS TO RESIDENTS

How can acquiring the perspective we are calling systems-informed professionalism benefit the resident? We will argue that this perspective gives residents a way to make sense of and to evaluate the world they are experiencing.

The resident lives in an organizational contex, and the influences arising from this context gives the resident clear signals about the priorities and values of the organization. Rightly or wrongly these signals shape the resident's view of the practice of medicine and the meaning of professionalism. We are referring here to the "hidden curriculum," which Fred Hafferty defines as a "set of influences that function at the level of organizational structure and culture."[27] Hafferty argues that this is where most of what is learned is learned, particularly the skills required to practice medicine and the values that the practice will embody.

The organization's purpose and the values associated with it determine the allocation decisions it makes. These decisions — how these resources are used — form the basis of an organization's structure, because the structure of any organization is comprised of the systems, processes, policies, and activities that enable the organization to fulfill its purpose — and they require resources in order to function — both human and technological.

Structure is thus part of the organization's culture, and both structure and culture inform the ethical climate of the organization. The ethical climate also reflects the beliefs of stakeholders about the organization's goals and values.[28] Thus, the structure and culture of any organization sets the stage for stakeholders' beliefs about what the organization represents. And, in the case of residency education, when a resident develops competence and then leaves the academic health center in which he or she trains, the resident might believe that the structure, goals, and values he or she sees, that the beliefs he or she encounters, are representative of the whole of "organized medicine." But there is ample evidence that there are differences among healthcare organizations, and that there may, in fact, be a gap between any healthcare organization's structure and culture and the goals and values espoused by many professional physician groups,[29] and this unfortunately also applies to academic health centers.[30]

Several chapters in this book have argued that the culture of the academic health center prevents or puts barriers in the path of resident's learning. For instance, both David Ozar and Evan

DeRenzo, in their respective chapters, discuss barriers the academic health center may place in the way of residency learning. They discuss how these barriers may prevent learning or blind the resident into accepting a "truth" about the practice of medicine or medical professionalism that may or may not correspond to the goals and values espoused by professional physician groups making up what we call "organized medicine." But systems-informed professionalism gives residents a framework in which they can ascertain what is really going on. Residents can use the framework to identify systems, to identify their purpose, the ways in which they achieve their purpose, and their effectiveness. Because residents are beginning to look at the ways a system achieves its purpose, they can identify roles and their function within the system. Residents can begin to identify when roles are not properly aligned or when function is misplaced. Residents can begin to identify gaps or shortfalls or misalignment in system effectiveness. And they can evaluate surrounding systems relative to their own goals and values.

This framework may benefit residents on practical and personal levels. On a practical level, it enables residents to understand roles and functions more clearly. It enables them to differentiate isolated events from system events — which may allow them to frame accountability issues appropriately. Furthermore, as residents move among hospitals and healthcare systems, it allows them to evaluate and compare systems, with an eye to improving their own practice. On a more personal level, it also allows residents to discern why there may be gap between the organization's culture and the values that they believe are appropriate to professionalism.

CONCLUSION

The managed-care movement, with its focus on cost-control, has been enormously frustrating to physicians. Physicians have seen their autonomy decreased; they have been asked to consider issues they traditionally have not been asked to consider; they have had to respond to managed care by creating structures of practice and relationships that they may not feel entirely comfortable with; they have had the regulations and requirements of practice increase while simultaneously facing decreasing reimbursement. So there are good reasons for physicians to be frustrated. Nevertheless, physicians are responsible to their profession. They contribute either positively or negatively to its evolution, and there is no doubt that the medical profession, the values associated with it, as well as its place in society, are evolving.

Prestigious organizations[31] and experts on healthcare[32] are insisting, and, in our opinion, rightly so, that the systems within which physicians work, not individuals, are the major culprits for inadequate care. Organizational systems are the embodiment of the goals and values of the organization, not of the individual. However, the ACGME suggests that individual physicians ought to accept at least partial responsibility for the development and improvement of these systems. There are accountability issues that must be addressed before this can be a reality — and responsibility without the power to effect appropriate change is always problematic. Outcomes associated with these issues will determine whether or not the ACGME mandates will add to the frustration of physicians or allow them more say in the design of systems that surround them and their patients. Regardless of the outcome, however, a perspective characterized by systems-informed professionalism will allow the individual physician to assess the construct and effectiveness of the systems which surround him or her. And surely, being able to adequately and appropriately assess these systems is the first step in the path to being able to help ensure that the healthcare systems of the future are designed to provide high quality, cost-effective care while reflecting the values associated with medical professionalism, which also include the values endorsed by society as appropriate to healthcare.

ACKNOWLEDGMENTS

We gratefully acknowledge the advice and comments of Bradford B. Worrall and Walter S. Davis in the preparation of this chapter. Donna Chen is supported in part by NIMH grant 1P20MH071897.

NOTES

1. *http://www.acgme.org/outcome/comp/compFull.asp*.
2. For a fuller explanation of the systems-informed professionalism framework, see chapter two.
3. R.S. Kaplan and D.P. Norton, *The Balanced Scorecard:*

Translating Strategy into Action (Boston, Mass.: Harvard Business School Press, 1996).

4. ACGME, see note 1 above.

5. T. Inui, *A Flag in the Wind: Educating for Professionalism in Medicine*, (Washington, D.C.: Association of American Medical Colleges, February 2003), 26.

6. Ibid., 26.

7. P.H. Werhane, *Moral Imagination and Management Decision Making*. (New York: Oxford University Press. 1999), 93.

8. Ibid.

9. Ibid.

10. Ibid. See also chapter five in Werhane, above.

11. P. Batalden et al., "General Competencies and Accreditation in Graduate Medical Education," *Health Affairs* 21, no. 5 (September-October 2002), 103-11. See also D. Leach, "Competence Is a Habit," *Journal of the American Assocition* 287, no. 2 (9 January 2002), 243-4; and G. Ogrinc et al., "A Framework for Teaching Medical Students and Residents about Practice-Based Learning and Improvement, Synthesized from a Literature Review," *Academic Medicine* 78, no. 7 (July 2003), 748-56.

12. H.L. Dreyfus, "What is Moral Maturity? A Phenomenological Account of the Development of Ethical Expertise," *istsocrates.berkeley.edu/~hdreyfus/rtf/Moral_ Maturity_8_90.rtf*, accessed 5 September 2005, also published as H. L. Dreyfus and S. E. Dreyfus, "What is Morality? A Phenomenological Account of the Development of Ethical Expertise," in *Universalism vs. Communitarianism,* ed. D. Rasmussen (Boston: MIT Press, 1990), 237-64.

13. Batalden et al., see note 11 above.

14. Ibid., 106.

15. Ibid.

16. The development of cynicism during undergraduate medical education is well documented, and it is likely that, in today's healthcare world, systems-related issues add significantly to the frustration and anger that contribute to the development of cynicism. Some training programs have experienced success in countering these effects. For examples of long-standing observations on cynicism, see for example, L.D. Eron, "The Effect of Medical Education on Attitudes: A Follow-up Study," *Journal of Medical Education* 33 (1958), 25-33; A.G. Rezler, "Attitude Changes During Medical School: A Review of the Literature," *Journal of Medical Education* 49 (1974): 1023-30; L. Kopelman, "Cynicism

Among Medical Students, *Journal of the American Medical Association* 250 (1183): 2006-10; and J. Coulehan and P. Williams, "Vanquishing Virtue: The Impact of Medical Education," *Academic Medicine* 76 (2001), 598-605. For examples of programs describing success in combating cynicism, see, for example, W.P. Roche, III, et al., "Medical Students' Attitudes in a PBL Curriculum: Trust, Altruism, and Cynicism," *Academic Medicine* 78, no. 4 (April 2003), 398-402.

17. As Batalden et. al. point out, physicians should learn to maintain an "involved response," in which physicians learn to "simply feel bad when a mistake is made and good when the right thing is done." Learning to manage this complex psychological response and using it as an aide to guide decision making and action continues during the residency training process and is further refined as one continues in practice. However, ultimately achieving an "involved response" first requires the ability to step back and disengage from the emotions in order to analyze the situation. As physicians develop, they will develop the ability to analyze a situation while remaining "involved." Batalden et al., see note 11 above.

18. This process can also been called "reflection on practice," which, with practice and experience, will become "reflection in practice," as the more experienced physician will be more able to use moral imagination and reflective practice during a conflict situation, rather than needing the time and space that less experienced physicians require. Although, when a situation is novel, even experienced physicians will need to disengage and create distance in time and space to "reflect on practice." As described above, this process entails learning skills and sensitivities that will continue to be refined during the residency training years and beyond. And, as described above, the systems-informed professionalism framework can help structure the process of moral imagination and reflection. Internalizing the framework provided by systems-informed professionalism is one step toward developing the mental model that will enable "reflection in practice." See, for example, D.M. Frankford, M.A. Patterson, and T.R.Konrad, "Transforming Practice Organizations to Foster Life-long Learning and Commitment to Medical Professionalism," *Academic Medicine* 75, no. 7 (July 2000): 708-17. (Frankford et al. call it "reflection on action" and "reflection in action.")

19. Batalden et al., see note 11 above, p. 106.

20. Ibid.

21. Ibid., 106.

22. T. Glick, "Viewpoint: Evidence Guided Education: Patients' Outcome Data Should Influence our Teaching Priorities," *Academic Medicine* 80, no. 2 (February 2005), 147-51.

23. R. Ziegelstein and N. Fieback, "'The Mirror" and 'The Village': A New Method for Teaching Practice Based Learning and Improvement and Systems Based Practice," *Academic Medicine* 79, no. 1 (January 2004) 83-88.

24. G. Dunnington and R. Williams, "Addressing the New Competencies for Residents' Surgical Training," *Academic Medicine* 78, no. 1 (2003), 14-21.

25. Ziegelstein and Fieback, see note 23 above.

26. Ibid.

27. F. W. Hafferty, "Beyond Curriculum Reform: Confronting Medicine's Hidden Curriculum," *Academic Medicine* 73, no. 4 (April 1998): 404.

28. We avoid the fine distinctions between the "culture school" and the "climate school" in the organization behavior literature by adopting Denison's position, that both address a common phenomenon that he views as the creation and influence of social contexts in organizations. The culture, the climate, and, more specifically, the ethical climate of an organization all relate to the social context of the organization, which includes the values and the assumptions on which individuals associated with an organization interact, carry out their activities, and make their decisions. See D.R. Denison, "What is the difference between organizational culture and organizational climate? A native's point of view on a decade of paradigm wars," *Academy of Management Review* 21 (1996): 619-54.

29. See note 16 above.

30. The Commonwealth Fund calls for medical education reform in the report "Training Tomorrow's Doctors." The report focuses on academic health centers (AHC), and addresses the role and responsibilities of the AHC, as well as offering practical guidance in the ways physicians should be schooled. "A Report of the Commonwealth Fund Task Force on Academic Health Centers: Training Tomorrow's Doctors. The Medical Education Mission of Academic Health Centers," 2002, *www.cmwf.org*, accessed August 2005.

31. Committee on Quality and Health Care in America, Institute of Medicine, *Crossing the Quality Chasm: A New Health System for the 21st Century* (Washington D.C.: National Acad-

emy Press, 2001).

32. A.C. Enthoven and L.A.Tollen, "Competition in Health Care: It takes Systems to Pursue Quality and Efficiency," *Health Affairs* (September 2005) *http://content. healthaffairs.org/cgi/content/abstract/hlthaff.w5.420,* accessed 7 September 2005. Also see S. Spear, "Fixing Health Care from the Inside, Today," *Harvard Business Review* (September 2005): 78-91.

11

The Challenges of a Residency Education Program for Competencies in Organizational Ethics

David T. Ozar

INTRODUCTION

Recently, the topic selected by the residents for their monthly "ethics rounds" session at Evanston Hospital (of Evanston Northwestern Healthcare, Evanston, Illinois) was the presence of fast-food restaurants and similar kinds of food offerings in the hospital cafeteria and cafeterias across the country. Given the high association between fast-food habits and insulin resistance and other health problems, the residents wanted to look at this issue. The resident who introduced the topic expressed both uncertainty about whether this could be counted as an ethics issue, and deep conviction that it raises important questions about the extent of physicians' and healthcare institutions' commitment to their patients' health.

The resident supported his conviction of the importance of the issue with a sample of the scientific literature on the link between fast-food habits with health problems[1] and an internet report of a Cleveland Clinic cardiovascular surgeon trying to get a fast-food restaurant out of the hospital.[2] But this resident and the other residents continued to express uncertainty about whether this should count as an ethical issue. In due course, I intervened to say that it was most assuredly an ethics issue, but of a sort that we were not accustomed to discuss in a direct way in our ethics rounds. It was an issue of organizational ethics, and it was not at all surprising that the residents were not sure if it "counted" as ethics, because residents' ethics education hardly ever addresses organizational ethics issues. As the leader of these ethics rounds sessions for 20 years, I have often pointed out the organizational components of the clinical ethics issues we have discussed. But residents are strongly predisposed by their training to see the organizational components of ethics questions as side issues, rather than as issues that are directly pertinent to their professional commitments as physicians.

This is why it is so important that competencies in organizational ethics are included among the educational outcomes for residency programs that are proposed in the long-term Outcome Project, recently initiated by the Accreditation Council for Graduate Medical Education (ACGME).[3] The overall purpose of the Outcome Project is to identify specific competencies as the principal educational outcomes of medical residency programs and to also focus attention on identifying appropriate modes of assessment, that is, concrete measures of the achievement of these competencies. To date, ACGME has identified six general areas of competency, and, within each area, a number of more specific competencies. Two of the six general areas, namely *professionalism* and *systems-based practice*, include competencies in the area of organizational ethics. The aim of this essay is to develop a more detailed account of educational outcomes for residents in the area of organizational ethics and to describe some of the specific challenges that will face educational and organizational leaders seeking to educate their residents effectively in organizational ethics.

To put this discussion in context, the other four general areas of competence identified by ACGME (included in the appendix to this volume) are: patient care, medical knowledge, practice-based learning and improvement, and interpersonal and communication skills. Within the general area of professionalism, the following are the specific competencies that include elements of organizational ethics:

> Residents must demonstrate a commitment to carrying out professional responsibilities, adherence to ethical principles, and sensitivity to a diverse patient population. Residents are expected to:

The Challenges of a Residency Education Program

- demonstrate respect, compassion, and integrity; a responsiveness to the needs of patients and society that supersedes self-interest; accountability to patients, society, and the profession; and a commitment to excellence and ongoing professional development
- demonstrate a commitment to ethical principles pertaining to provision or withholding of clinical care, confidentiality of patient information, informed consent, and business practices
- demonstrate sensitivity and responsiveness to patients' culture, age, gender, and disabilities[4]

Within the general area of systems-based practice, these are the specific competencies that include elements of organizational ethics:

Residents must demonstrate an awareness of and responsiveness to the larger context and system of health care and the ability to effectively call on system resources to provide care that is of optimal value. Residents are expected to:

- understand how their patient care and other professional practices affect other health care professionals, the health care organization, and the larger society and how these elements of the system affect their own practice
- know how types of medical practice and delivery systems differ from one another, including methods controlling health care costs and allocating resources
- practice cost-effective health care and resource allocation that does not compromise quality of care
- advocate for quality patient care and assist patients in dealing with system complexities
- know how to partner with health care managers and health care providers to assess, coordinate, and improve health care and know how these activities can affect system performance[5]

PART ONE: EDUCATIONAL OUTCOMES

Outcomes-based curriculum design begins by answering the "outcomes question," namely: "As a result of the proposed learning experience, what is it that the learner will be able to do or to do better, that he or she could not do or could not do as well before?" One important goal of the ACGME Outcome Project is to identify the principal learning outcomes of medical residency programs. However, it is a mark of effective outcomes-based curriculum design that the outcome or competency is stated in such a way that another question, the "assessment question," can be answered clearly and concretely as well. The "assessment question" is: "How will you be able to tell if the learner has achieved the intended learning outcome?"[6]

It is an eventual goal of the Outcome Project that concrete, effective methods of assessment of its proposed competencies will eventually be identified or developed. But it is a weakness of the competencies currently identified by ACGME that few of them are currently stated in such a way that the "assessment question" can be answered clearly, much less concretely. So the ACGME's sense that there is still a lot of work to be done is clearly correct. While this essay will not attempt to complete the task of answering the "assessment question" for all of the educational outcomes discussed here, it is hoped that, for most of the outcomes discussed, it will be clear from their formulation how, at least in general terms, learners' achievement of these outcomes could be assessed.

One way to clarify the competencies/outcomes proposed by ACGME is to compare them with, and then to parse them in turn into, appropriate subcompetencies in terms of the four components of the moral life that a psychologist of moral development, James Rest, employed to illuminate the processes of moral growth and moral education.[7] These four components are:

1. *Awareness of or sensitivity to* what is ethically significant in a situation and of the alternative courses of action available to respond to it;
2. *The reasoning and reflective skills* needed to reach, from the ethical data available in a situation, a sound ethical judgment about how to act, that is, which of the identified alternatives ought to be done;
3. *Motivation* to perform the action that is identified in a sound ethical judgment as the action that ought to be done; and
4. *Implementation*, that is, the emotional and practical abilities needed to carry out the course of action identified as what ought to be done.[8]

For example, in the ethics rounds session mentioned above, one reason that the residents were uncertain how to formulate their issue as an ethics question was a deficit in *awareness*. They had no idea of the organizational structures involved in making decisions about food service contracts in the hospital and how and by whom competing bids for these contracts are evaluated and decided upon. In addition, the residents had no trouble imagining people making food decisions in the hospital cafeteria and being drawn to fast-food options out of habit or time considerations. They also could easily imagine people making healthier choices if the fast-food options were not present. But their imaginations were much more limited about how the fast-food options came to be offered in the cafeteria in the first place.[9] The residents were also unable to readily identify practical courses of action that they themselves might take to have an impact on these evaluations and decisions, another deficit in awareness. The proper educational response to these deficits is an effort to enhance residents' awareness of the organizational systems within which they operate, both the systems of their own institution and those of the larger society within which the hospital itself must function.

Assessing the effectiveness of such efforts will ordinarily involve eliciting relevant narratives. For example, asking residents to describe how food service decisions are made in their hospital, and by whom, and on what bases. They would also need to be able to describe courses of action by which interested parties might represent to institutional decision makers the considerations that these parties judge are being given inadequate weight in food service decisions.

In addition, even when solid ethical *reasoning and reflective skills* yield sound ethical judgments and *motivation* for organizational change is strong, residents and many other organizational subgroups often experience significant emotional and practical barriers to *implementing* actions that will practically impact organizational structures. Two such barriers will be discussed in detail in part two of this chapter, and a general framework for educational interventions outlined in part three. But the initial lesson is that, without focused educational attention on residents' awareness of how they might address ethical issues at the organizational level, few of them will leave residency with any sense of how to implement their ethical judgments about organizational ethics.

It might be objected at this point that residents have rarely had enough experience, both in sheer quantity and especially in terms of the scope or breadth of their experience, for their involvement in organizational matters to be something that might be expected or even desired. But in fact, these men and women will soon be independently practicing physicians, that is, persons of genuine power within the American healthcare system. To be sure, their effective power within particular institutions will typically begin small and grow only over time. But it would be a serious educational mistake to think that *leadership* is not something they should be educated for while they are residents. Physicians are the dominant teachers/shapers of American healthcare, whether they are comfortable in this role or not. These young physicians will therefore be leaders, bearers of power, before very long, so *leadership* is a fifth category of ethical activity that needs educational attention during residency, particularly from the perspective of organizational ethics. That is, now is the time to begin to train these young physicians in the ethical use of their power as physicians.

The competencies relevant to organizational ethics in the ACGME section on systems-based practices, cited above, do not only mention that residents should "know" and "understand" about organizations, and that they should "advocate" and "practice" (that is, personally) accordingly. The competencies also, at least once, hold that residents should "advocate." Such advocacy is *leadership,* and there is little reason to think that residents will learn how to exercise ethical advocacy during their residency years unless there is a deliberate and explicit learning outcome in organizational ethics leadership for residency programs.

PART TWO: THE BARRIERS

Why is there little reason to think that residents will become skilled in exercising ethical advocacy and leadership during their residency years unless there is a deliberate and explicit learning outcome in organizational ethics leadership for residency programs? Why is it that, without focused educational attention on how residents can practically implement their concerns about organizational ethical issues, few of them will leave residency with any sense of how to do this? Why is it that residents are typically unable to identify practical courses of action that they might take to have an impact on organizational evaluations and decisions?

There are two parts to the answer to these questions. The first concerns the powerlessness of residents within the organizations where they learn and practice medicine. This impacts their awareness and also constitutes an emotional barrier to implementation. The second concerns a widespread poverty of conceptual tools for articulating and discussing organizational ethics issues, not only among residents, but among those who teach them and among healthcare professionals generally—and in fact throughout the larger community. This barrier also impacts awareness and reduces residents' ability to conceive of organizational concerns as legitimate ethical issues. Each of these barriers needs to be described in more detail before relevant educational interventions can be described, even at a general level.

It should be clear to anyone who is familiar with hospital residency programs that residents are not powerful within institutions. It is true that residents provide a great deal of the day-to-day medical care received by a teaching hospital's patients, and the presence of residents in a hospital means that most medical judgments made there are made by, and confirmed within, a group of trained experts, rather than judgments made solo by single practitioners. But this does not mean that residents have much power within institutions, and their need to successfully survive performance reviews at many levels and at the hands of many physicians and other persons of power reinforces their sense of dependence on "the way things are" at the institution.

Residents' lack of institutional power and their constant dependence on those who have power within institutions are more than experiential realities in the lives of residents. They soon become part of each new resident's self-concept. Indeed, the institutional powerlessness of residents is such an obvious reality and so readily absorbed into residents' self-concepts that most new residents arrive at the beginning of residency already formed in the view that they are powerless within their institution; and their institutions' centers of power almost always oblige with powerful reinforcements of this predisposition from day one.

Further, the impact of this disposition on their imaginations is substantial, especially in very busy people who have little time for introspection. Organizations are conservative in the root sense of that word; they exist to provide stability to certain categories of social relationships, preserving patterns of social interaction that have worked in the past. Therefore, even persons and subgroups who have some power within organizations recognize that organizational change does not occur easily. But those who are disposed to view themselves as powerless, as the ones over whom institutional power is exercised rather than as ones who possess it, are even more prone to see their organization as immoveable and are typically very clear that, even if it can change, such change will not be initiated by them. The ability of residents to imagine their organization as otherwise than it is in some respect is sharply reduced by their sense of themselves as powerless within it.

For the same reason, and with added emphasis because their performance is constantly under scrutiny, residents find it hard to imagine how they might initiate a change in their organization. Even in these residency programs in which residents do have ready access to a department chief or chair, it is that person, not the resident, who has the power to make things happen. The paths of power are not open to residents in any obvious way, and this sharply limits their awareness of the actions they might take to address organizational issues that they become aware of. In fact, teaching hospitals are so dependent on the medical services provided by residents that residents might actually be able, if they could act as a unified group, to wield genuine power within an institution. But, for most residents, this possibility exists only in the abstract, because of their continual dependence on positive reviews by their superiors; it has little practical impact on their views of issues in organizational ethics.

The second barrier is a conceptual barrier, a widespread poverty of conceptual tools for articulating and discussing organizational ethics issues. Day-in, day-out, most people in our society seem to look on organizations as if they were vast machines whose activities are composed, from an ethical point of view, entirely of the actions of individual human persons. The idea that an organization is actually, in many important respects, quite similar to an individual human decision maker is simply not given much consideration. And this means that, when ethical issues arise within the life of an organization, the tendency is to see them solely as the ethical issues of certain individuals. Frequently this means that the important aspects of the issue will be missed, because very important elements of it will be left unconceptualized and, therefore, unexamined.[10]

The Challenges of a Residency Education Program

Of course, there is significant scholarly literature on organizations, organizational behavior, and organizational development, much of which looks upon organizations as unitary entities that face alternative courses of action, engage in deliberation about them, make choices and act accordingly, and confront the results of their choices. That is, organizations are often viewed as morally responsible actors who are capable of actions that are either ethical or unethical.[11] It is also the case that, in ordinary speech, people do often speak of corporations and other organizations as if they were ethically similar to individual humans. Corporations and other organizations are often said to have acted unethically or ethically, to have failed in their responsibilities or to have fulfilled them, to have rights deserving of respect or to have rights whose moral import is less than other parties' rights in a situation. But these patterns of speech do not trigger a "deep" conceptualization of organizations like hospitals and health systems as ethically significant actors whose structures, systems, roles, and relations deserve specific ethical examination, which examination is what is meant by "organizational ethics."

But, as the philosopher Henri Bergson is reported to have said, it is extremely difficult to notice something that one has no concept for. The first result, for our residents, of our society's poverty of conceptual tools for articulating and discussing organizations as ethically significant decision makers, actors, and bearers of responsibility for their actions is to sharply reduce residents' awareness of organizational matters as ethical issues. Hence the residents' uncertainty during ethics rounds, that the issue of serving fast food in the restaurant should count as an ethics issue. The second result of the poverty of conceptual tools for organizational ethics is that residents lack understanding of the components of organizational action, and therefore can ordinarily conceive of organizational change only in terms of "revolution," which they rightly consider unlikely.

A richer conceptual repertoire would not only enhance their awareness of the ethical and unethical activities of their hospital, but enable them to identify ways in which specific structures, systems, roles, or relationships might change without an overthrow of the whole institution. For example, they might be able to imagine how the institution's core values have to be ranked by those who make decisions about food service contracts, because these values cannot all be maximally achieved in any of the available bids from vendors. Or they might be able to imagine how a conversation about these values with the director of purchasing might lead to the formation of a residents' committee on healthy food that might advise the director of purchasing. Perhaps an alliance with the hospital's chief nutritionist might be forged, or with sympathetic souls on the hospital's staff of attending physicians.

PART THREE: A GENERAL INSTRUCTIONAL FRAMEWORK ("THE CURRICULUM")

In most residency programs, it would be an educational revolution if the current program of clinical ethics discussions, akin to the ethics rounds sessions described above, were to be supplemented with a program of organizational ethics rounds. But, if competencies in organizational ethics are important — and they are — then something like this minimum is needed. Given the significant barriers to residents' becoming effective thinkers in organizational ethics that were just noted, it is foolhardy to think that such competencies are going to be achieved without considerable, focused educational effort. Moreover, to be truly portable to the residents' eventual practice situation, such a program should include not only issues that are currently in the lives of residents and their patients, but should also include issues that arise within the broader social and economic setting within which their institution must function—and within which, before too long, the residents, as independent professionals, will function as well.

Even apart from a more formal curriculum, organizational ethics rounds could enable instructors to provide residents with a basic conceptual framework about organizations and organizational ethics, to facilitate open discussion of issues in the hospital that are important to the residents, and to model and assist them in careful ethical reflection on concrete, alternative actions that might be taken. That is, such organizational ethics rounds could, like the clinical ethics rounds that have some currency in residency programs today, enhance awareness, enrich reasoning and reflective skills, address the barriers that hinder implementation, and foster leadership, with a specific focus on competencies in organizational ethics.

But it is worthwhile to formulate, at least in general terms, the elements of a more complete curriculum in organizational ethics, both as a goal that concerned residency programs might aim at, and as a guide to the most important elements that should be incorporated, in one way or another, into the conversational setting of organizational ethics rounds, if that is the most extensive educational effort that can be mustered in this area.

ELEMENT ONE: SOCIAL ANALYSIS

Intended outcome: To enhance organizational awareness, in general (through relevant concepts), and in regard to the particular issues examined.

1. The general structure of organizations, especially the role of mission and core organizational values, organizational fact-finding and decision-making systems, and so forth.
2. The structure of the hospital (and the healthcare system, if appropriate), especially its mission and core values, its fact-finding and decision-making systems, its internal structures and power relationships, et cetera.
3. The organizational structure of the particular issue, especially who are the relevant institutional decision makers, what facts they work with, what alternative courses of action or alternative policies they have considered, the specific value judgments involved in the issue (and in previous decisions about the issue if appropriate), other concerned constituencies, et cetera.

ELEMENT TWO: SOCIAL IMAGINATION

Intended outcome: To enhance awareness of how the organization might be, in general, and in the particular issues examined.

1. Imaging the particular situation otherwise: widely, vividly, creatively, and articulating these images for others.
2. Reality testing: Would the imagined reconstructions of the particular situation work for the persons who live in and/or use them, independent of the likelihood of their being implemented? (For example: Would they depend on a massive infusion of resources that would shut down another unit? Would they require heroic dedication on the part of too many ordinary people? And so on).
3. Imagine the institution otherwise, in ways that would make implementation of the particular reconstructions (at least the

realistic ones) institutionally plausible in terms of the reconstructed organizational mission/values/ systems/structures/ roles that might replace those of the current institution.

ELEMENT THREE: SOCIAL ETHICAL REFLECTION
Intended outcome: Enhanced *ethical* reasoning and reflective skills, applied specifically to particular organizational issues.

1. Evaluate the (realistic) imagined alternatives in comparison with what is the case,
2. Using the existing mission and core values of the institution,
3. Together with other conceptual tools for ethical evaluation of social systems, for example, concepts of justness, solidarity, collective good, collective agency, harm/benefit to various constituencies ("stakeholders"), et cetera.
4. Determine whether "deep" institutional change is what ought to take place, that is, that the ethically best course of action will require changes in structure within the institution or, more deeply, changes in mission and/or core organizational values.
5. Formulate this reflection in favor of one organizational course of action and share it with others for their evaluation of its strengths and weaknesses as ethical reasoning.

ELEMENT FOUR: IMPLEMENTATION STRATEGIES
Intended outcome: Enhanced awareness of possible personal action, assist implementation both practically and in relation to the emotional impact of powerlessness, that is, courage in place of fear, and hopefulness in place of hopelessness for change.

1. Examine, with imagination, what is possible within the existing "chain of command."
2. Examine, with imagination, what is possible through professional solidarity within the residents' own group.
3. Examine, with imagination, what is possible through professional solidarity with the attending physicians as collaborators or allies.
4. Examine, with imagination, what is possible through professional solidarity with other groups of professionals in the institution, et cetera.

5. Other possibilities: Avenues outside the institution (do the values at stake in the particular issue justify considering "whistle-blowing," et cetera?).

ELEMENT FIVE: THE RISKS OF IMPLEMENTATION AND THE PROPER ROLE OF ORGANIZATIONAL COURAGE

Intended outcome: Enhanced ethical reasoning and reflective skills, applied specifically to alternative modes of organizational intervention in relation to the particular issue under examination.

1. Realistically assess the extent and burdens of residents' institutional powerlessness.
2. Realistically assess the risks to individuals and groups if action is taken in this case.
3. Realistically weigh the values, benefits, and burdens, et cetera, that are at stake in the particular situation for all those affected by it.
4. Reflect on the ethics of institutional conscientious disobedience.

PART FOUR: THE ROLE OF ORGANIZATIONAL ETHICS LEADERS AND EDUCATORS

Those with the formal task of instructing residents in organizational ethics will need to apply their educational skills to lead the residents to the achievement of these competencies in ways that are, in one respect, very familiar. Effective instruction in most of what is included in the first four curricular elements identified in part three of this chapter will involve the same teaching strategies that are familiar from the teaching of clinical ethics to residents. While the subject matter is different because the intended outcomes — that is, competencies — are different, instructors will need the same skill at formulating ethical arguments in close, articulate detail to model the various approaches to ethical thinking for learners and to guide them in applying these skills to particular ethical issues. Although ethical thinking about social systems involves some concepts — for example, concepts of justness, solidarity, collective good, collective agency, harm/benefit to various constituencies ("stakeholders"), and so forth, that are not as commonly employed in clinical ethics issues, the basic approaches to ethical reflection in which these concepts are employed are the same.

Even in regard to the fifth element — weighing risks and reflecting on the courage needed to do what is right — those who teach clinical ethics will be in fairly familiar emotional territory because so many of the clinical ethical issues that residents need to discuss include their relationship to an attending, or, occasionally, some other person on whose authority or power the resident is dependent. But because organizational ethics issues are so rarely identified as such in the clinical setting, and also because the barriers discussed in part two of this chapter are so significant in the lives of residents, both the content and the emotions of the fifth element will require the instructor's special attention if the intended competencies are to be achieved. The instructor in organizational ethics must be able to be both highly imaginative and at the same time thoroughly practical about "imagining otherwise" about alternative ways in which particular issues might be approached, about possible avenues of institutional intervention within the "chain of command," about possible collaborations and allies outside the chain of command, about possible reconstructions of the structures, systems, roles, and relations within the organization, and even about possible reconstructions of the organization's mission and core values. If it is possible that there is a place where a rich imagination is even more valuable than in the teaching of clinical ethics to professional caregivers, the teaching of organizational ethics to professional caregivers is it.

There is one respect in which instruction in organizational ethics appears very similar to instruction in clinical ethics at first look, but proves to be significantly different when the matter is examined at greater depth. This concerns the ethics instructor as role model, that is, as modeling leadership in organizational ethics. In all education, but especially in professional formation and in ethics education, modeling is by far the most potent shaper of learners. Even in formal classrooms, at least as much is learned by the learners from the conduct of the instructor, in relation to the subject matter and in relation to the learners, and from the instructor's observed personal conduct, as is learned through the teacher's work with the formal curriculum. This is even truer in the clinical setting, whether the topic is clinical ethics or organizational ethics, because the instructor's

The Challenges of a Residency Education Program

acceptance into the clinical setting as an instructor by those in charge unavoidably commends him or her to the residents as someone modeling what they are to learn.

It is therefore important to comment, in closing, on the absolute necessity of persons in the residents' lives who will model organizational ethics reflection and leadership, to include, but hopefully not be limited to, those who are formally assigned to instruct residents in organizational ethics. Only by observing respected physicians and others in positions of respect, who actively engage in imagining otherwise, evaluating carefully, and acting appropriately in matters of organizational ethics, will residents come to value acquiring the capacities and skills identified above. And only by observing these competencies actively exercised, that is, modeled by persons whom they respect, will residents begin to absorb these competencies into their own personalities as patterns of awareness, reflection, and conduct.

This is why those who have been given the formal task of instructing residents in organizational ethics must themselves be models of these kinds of awareness, reflection, and conduct, and they must obviously be comfortably articulate about each of these activities. Of particular importance will be a willingness on the part of teachers in this area to address frankly with the residents the fact of the residents' institutional powerlessness, the typical impact of this fact on residents' self-image and imaginations, the risks of growth of awareness and reflection in a setting in which prudence may sometimes — with good ethical reason — suggest restraint rather than overt action, and the real risks that may accompany residents' actions for organizational change. To attempt to instruct residents in organizational ethics without candor about these aspects of residents' daily circumstances would significantly undermine the educational enterprise.

Finally, as a natural companion to the frankness about powerlessness and risk mentioned above, and as an unavoidable part of the modeling that is an essential part of teaching organizational ethics, the organizational ethics instructor must be willing to model professional solidarity with the residents in their organizational ethics concerns. At a minimum this will mean treating them in significant measure as peers, fellow physicians committed to the same values individually and collectively, even while finding mutually acceptable ways to live out the unavoidable differences in station, power, and experience. It will also sometimes mean accepting a role as adviser to the residents, individually or as a group, as they consider possible actions aimed at changing the institution for ethical reasons. In these respects, there is a strong analogy to what modeling good clinical ethics with the residents will require.

But in the case of organizational ethics, it may also mean that the instructor has to both determine thoughtfully whether or not to stand with residents in opposition to the institution, should this happen, and to share his or her decision and the reflections leading to it openly and honestly with the residents. Precisely because organizational ethics is about the ethics of social relations and the systems that embody them, one cannot be a teacher of organizational ethics and model the awareness, reflection, and conduct this implies, without deliberate attention to the particular social relation that exists between teacher and student, especially when both are members of the same profession. Examination of the ethics of that relationship and its potential implications for the instructor's relationship to the institution will be a necessary complement to the other educational skills needed to assist residents in achieving competencies in organizational ethics.

CONCLUSION

The ACGME is to be admired for acknowledging that the full formation of medical professionals cannot be accomplished without attention to the ethics of the organizations within which physicians necessarily practice. The current language of the Outcome Project only hints at the depth and scope of the educational outcomes that attention to organizational ethics requires. The aim of this essay has been to expand that vision and reflect on the challenges that will be faced by those who take it seriously, not only of those in charge of the ACGME Outcome Project, but of all those who teach residents and value their learning what they need to be fully ethical members of the medical profession.

ACKNOWLEDGMENT

An earlier version of this chapter appeared in *Organizational Ethics: Healthcare, Business, and Policy*, volume 2, no.1 (Spring

2005). ©2005, University Publishing Group. Used with permission. All rights reserved.

NOTES

1. M.A. Pereira et al., "Fast-food habits, weight gain, and insulin resistance (the CARDIA study): 15-year prospective analysis," *Lancet* 365, no. 9464 (1 January 2005): 36-42.

2. "The Cleveland Clinic battles with McDonald's over fast foods in hospitals," *www.newstarget.com/003915.html*, accessed 7 February 2005.

3. The ACGME website at *www.acgme.org/outcome* includes a number of Outcome Project documents, including the most recent version of the proposed competencies and some sample indications of assessment tools. There is, at this stage, nothing close to a mandate regarding assessment tools.

4. See *www.acgme.org/outcome/comp/refProf1.asp*.

5. Ibid.

6. Two fairly accessible resources on outcomes-based curriculum design have been useful in the development of this essay. Both of these focus their examples on primary and secondary education, but without in the least diminishing thereby their usefulness for curriculum design in postgraduate education. L.A. Ozar, *Creating a Curriculum That Works: A Guide to Outcomes-Centered Curriculum Decision-Making* (Washington, D.C.: National Catholic Educational Association, 1994), and G. Wiggins and J. McTighe, *Understanding by Design* (Alexandria, Va.: Association for Supervision and Curriculum Development, 1998).

7. J.R. Rest, "The Major Components of Morality," in *Morality, Moral Behavior, and Moral Development*, ed. W. Kurtines and J. Gewirtz (New York: Wiley, 1984); also J.R. Rest, "Background: Theory and Research," in *Moral Development in the Professions*, ed. J.R. Rest and D. Narvaez (Hillsdale, N.J.: Lawrence Erlbaum, 1994), 1-26, and J.R. Rest et al., *Postconventional Moral Thinking: A Neo-Kohlbergian Approach* (Hillsdale, N.J.: Lawrence Erlbaum, 1999).

8. This interpretation of Rest's four components of moral development and its application to formal ethics education is developed in detail in: D.T. Ozar, "Learning Outcomes For Ethics Across the Curriculum Programs," *Teaching Ethics* 2 (2001): 1-27, also available at *http://www.luc.edu/ethics/03150outcomes_teaching.shtml*.

9. On the role of expanded imagination in enhancing ethical reflection see, M. Johnson, *Moral Imagination: Implications of Cognitive Science for Ethics* (Chicago, Ill.: University of Chicago Press, 1993), and P.H. Werhane, *Moral Imagination and Management Decision-Making* (New York: Oxford University Press, Ruffin Series in Business Ethics, 1999).

10. A useful introduction to the concepts of organizational ethics in healthcare organizations will be found in D.T. Ozar et al., *Organizational Ethic in Health Care: A Framework for Ethical Decision-Making by Provider Organizations* (Chicago, Ill.: American Medical Association Institute of Ethics, 2000), *http://www.ama-assn.org/ama/upload/mm/369/organizational ethics.pdf*.

11. Some philosophers have held that human collectives invariably lack such characteristics as would justify holding collectives accountable for their actions rather than (or in addition to) holding the individuals within the organizations accountable, so such entities' actions could not be justifiably held to be either ethical or unethical. One of the best known is J. Ladd, "Morality and the Ideal of Rationality in Formal Organizations," *Monist* 54 (1970): 488-516. See also M. Valesquez, "Why Corporations Are Not Morally Responsible for Anything They Do," *Business and Professional Ethics Journal* 2 (1983): 1-18.

12

The Patient's Perspective in the ACGME Systems-Based Practice Competency

Walter S. Davis

INTRODUCTION

In developing the six General Competencies, the ACGME used a research and collaborative review process that included a cross-section of key stake holders in healthcare, with representation from the medical profession, residents, medical educators, employers of physicians, the U.S. government, healthcare quality monitors, community health providers, society-at-large as typified by a private foundation, and of course, patients. (The General Competencies are included in full in an appendix to this volume.) The patient perspective is obviously important for all six of the competency areas, but it is perhaps the systems-based competency that is the least intuitive of these in terms of how the patient perspective is important. Because the quality of healthcare provided by the generation of physicians trained under the new guidelines will ultimately be judged by patients, it is useful to examine the role of the patient perspective in these new competencies, and explore how the patient perspective might be included in residency education.

In this chapter, I begin by looking generally at what the ACGME competencies might, and might not, mean for patients. I then look closely at the systems-based practice competency, specify how the patient perspective is important to its five elements as set out by the ACGME, and outline what this might mean for the physician-patient relationship as we attempt to educate a new cohort of physicians to take the "broad view" of healthcare and apply it to their practice. I then present two patient perspectives — opposing ends of a spectrum — from my own experience working with patients within various healthcare systems. Finally, I offer some suggestions as to how the competency-based model of residency program accreditation might assess the new generation of physicians' ability to act as patient advocates in the face of ever-increasing calls for systems-based practice and system-wide accountability — which is a key component of professionalism in systems-based practice.

WHERE IS THE PATIENT PERSPECTIVE IN THE NEW ACCREDITATION PROCESS?

First off, we must admit that patients are unlikely to be aware of any changes in the accreditation system for residency training programs at any point. The dynamics of healthcare are such that the perspective of patients is shaped by a multitude of factors, and we will probably not be able to discern to what degree the changes in patients' perspectives are due to changes in physician education like the ACGME Outcome Project. One can assume that all patients would be in favor of an accreditation program for medical residencies that assures competency in key areas — indeed, most patients probably assume that such a program is already in place — but it is less clear how patients might view the individual elements of competent practice.

Also, it is important to remember the ACGME competencies do not, in themselves, represent something completely new. Many aspects of the six competencies can be found in recent deliberations about medical education. Over the last five to 10 years, many of the curriculum changes in medical education have reflected these deliberations, which include stressing the importance of the patient perspective.[1] The ACGME Outcome Project represents the next step in a long journey of re-examining the process by which we educate and train physicians. It brings these competencies together, for the first time, as a requirement for residency training. And, as the ACGME points out, the important change is in the accreditation process itself — a change from a "minimal-threshold model," which identifies whether a residency program has the potential to educate residents, to a "competency-based model," which examines whether the program is actually educating them. The new emphasis is on "educational outcomes," which, the ACGME is quick to point out, should not be confused with clinical outcomes. Clinical outcomes, the ACGME says, certainly can and should be used as educational outcomes for several of the General Competencies, but they are not the only educational outcomes of residency education, and are not the whole picture.[2]

Why the focus on educational outcomes? As the ACGME points out, they are late in the outcomes movement, essentially "playing catch up" with other accrediting bodies in the health professions, education, and business that have focused on educational outcomes since the 1980s, when the U.S. Department of Education mandated a move towards greater use of outcome assessment in professional accreditation. Also, because the U.S. system of medical education is heavily reliant upon public funding, medical educators are under increasing pressure to show that they are preparing competent physicians to meet the healthcare needs of the public that supports them.

WHERE IS THE PATIENT PERSPECTIVE IN THE SYSTEMS-BASED COMPETENCY REQUIREMENT?

The ACGME guidelines divide the systems-based practice competency into five specific expectations. I discuss the patient perspective in each of the five specific expectations and explore ways to ensure that this perspective is a part of teaching and assessing that expectation.

1. *Residents should understand how their patient care and other professional practices affect other health care professionals, the health care organization, and the larger society and how these elements of the system affect their own practice.* Most patients are aware of the large number of individuals, medical professionals, and others involved in today's healthcare environment. While they may not understand the specific interaction between all of these elements, it is reasonable to assume that they expect their physician to be able to accurately represent the facts of their medical status to others in the system. In this re-

gard, accurate and timely documentation of the medical services recommended and provided would be an example of a basic competency from the perspective of most patients. Much of healthcare reimbursement depends on the specifics of documentation, and having residents understand how this documentation affects communication with other professionals, and, ultimately, the quality of care provided to the patient, is essential. Patients may need to be reassured that their physician is communicating with other professionals and the organization at large in a way that benefits them and their healthcare, and it will most likely be up to physicians themselves to provide this reassurance.

There are certainly many ways that resident educators can incorporate this competency goal into their training programs. For example, they might have residents participate in a "case follow-up" two or three times a year, in which they would review, in a somewhat "forensic" fashion, a patient they had treated early in the course of the disease or complaint. This would involve using the medical record to review their own documentation and see how it was interpreted and used by other professionals, seeing where the patient ended up after leaving their care, identifying problem areas in the "system" and where they might have been able to improve, and seeing how billing and insurance coverage for the overall treatment course and individual procedures played out. The idea would be that residents would get a sense of where they, as physicians, fall in the chain of events, and their role in shaping the quality of an individual's healthcare experience.

2. Residents should know how types of medical practice and delivery systems differ from one another, including methods of controlling health care costs and allocating resources. While most of the interaction between the patient and the physician should be focused on listening to the patient's complaint, providing information about the plan to evaluate the complaint, and, finally, communicating with the patient regarding diagnosis, treatment, and follow-up, in today's healthcare environment patients and their physicians are also required to exchange information about the "system" within which the patient is receiving care. The physician may need to explain how his or her practice is set up, what to expect when another physician is covering, and how referrals and diagnostic work-up are handled. The patient, in turn, may need to explain how his or her insurance coverage might affect the recommendations of the physician and the subsequent treatment course. This is particularly important when the treatment in question is difficult, expensive, experimental, rarely recommended, or all of the above. In most healthcare organizations, there are explicit, ongoing initiatives to control costs for the most common, expensive, or unpredictable conditions, but an individual patient may not understand how those efforts will affect his or her care. The physician is the link between information about the scientifically based clinical condition and the patient's perception of the disease experience. The "system's" response to, and support of, the patient is only one part of that experience, but probably one in which the physician should be intimately involved.

For this competency, residents would need some basic didactic efforts simply to explain the structure of various healthcare delivery systems, preferably ones in which they, as residents, actually participate in. This won't always be possible, since some residency programs only operate within a single facility or system; in these cases, larger systems in the area or systems in which residents in the field are likely to work after residency would be reasonable. This might take the form of having the medical director or other administrator for the health system present an overview of the system and how it's arranged, but the didactic experience could then be enriched by having the administrator explain how, specifically, healthcare costs are controlled and resources allocated within the system. This will involve a level of "institutional" honesty and disclosure that might make some administrators uncomfortable, but in this respect we may see the ACGME competency requirements actually have an effect on organizational ethics as it applies to healthcare systems. If we continue to exclude residents from the difficult or controversial decisions that are made in our delivery systems, we cannot and should not expect them to transition smoothly into their careers and become effective members of healthcare system "teams."

This competency might also include specific didactic efforts aimed at the more common government-sponsored third-party payers such as Medicare and Medicaid. Residents obviously take care of large numbers of patients covered under these systems, but often leave residency not understanding how the programs work, or how their practice is affected by changes in these systems. This type of didactic content would be particularly useful, and perhaps more compelling for residents, if it focused on how federally sponsored programs operate for treatment and procedures within the residents' medical specialty. A general overview of the programs might be appropriate to begin with, but presentations with titles like "The Medicaid Patient with a Chronic Psychiatric Disorder" or "The Patient with COPD and Medicaid" are probably more useful in the long run. This type of educational content not only teaches the specifics of the programs, but gives residents a closer, more personal look into the experiences of their individual patients in the healthcare system.

3. *Residents should practice cost-effective health care and resource allocation that does not compromise quality of care.* Patients, by definition, are experiencing some degree of suffering, and are necessarily focused on getting appropriate and effective treatment for their medical problem. They want to believe that their physician's priority is the quality of care, and they may not be prepared to consider cost-effectiveness as a goal, however subordinate, in their care. This competency, then, not only requires that residents learn to provide high-quality, cost-effective care, but also to learn the communication skills necessary to help patients understand that, while the quality of care is the primary goal, cost-effectiveness is important and will be evident in the "system" in which their care is based.

Perhaps the simplest and most direct way to teach this competency would be to use some of the "success stories" that were reviewed by the ACGME committee that formulated the competencies. One of the references cited by the ACGME for "Systems-Based Practice" is an article that appeared in 1998 in the *Journal of the American Medical Association,* which suggested that a systems-based approach to changing a medical service resulted in improved resource use and did not affect clinical outcomes or the satisfaction of patients, faculty, and housestaff.[3] These types of didactic efforts are particularly effective if they contain the direct perspectives of the patients involved, such as patient satisfaction surveys, individual patient "exit interviews," et cetera. Knowing at least the basics of these success stories provides physicians with information they can use as they participate in improving care in their own systems, and allows them to know how, specifically, the patient perspective can be used in these efforts to assure quality care.

4. *Residents should advocate for quality patient care and assist patients in dealing with system complexities.* Advocating for quality care requires good communication skills — first at the level of physician-to-patient — but also with other healthcare professionals. In this respect, much of the work done to teach communication skills in medical schools may have prepared residents to act as patient advocates. But effective advocacy also requires that physicians have enough knowledge of the system so that they know where to aim their advocacy efforts. This compentency involves substantial interplay with the other systems-based competencies. Patients want their physicians to understand, and sometimes explain and interpret, the systems in which they receive healthcare, but ultimately they expect their physicians to be their advocates in the healthcare world.

For this competency, it will be necessary to teach residents some of the basic skills in advocating for patients within the most common kinds of healthcare systems. One specific place to start is to teach negotiation skills that are useful when doing the classic "peer-to-peer" review — when a patient has been denied insurance coverage for a treatment or procedure by a third-party payer. It is helpful, for instance, for residents to know that many of the physicians who work as case reviewers for healthcare organizations also see themselves as patient advocates, and that focusing on the positive patient outcome that is likely to result from the treatment, rather than on attempting to be a mouthpiece for the patient's anger and dissatisfaction, is more likely to result in a successful appeal. Not all appeals will be successful, of course, so teaching residents how and why to "pick their battles" is an important skill. Residents will most likely benefit from role-playing these scenarios with experienced physician mentors to learn to mount the most convincing arguments using medical fact, rather than the language of confrontation and perceived injustice; they should also, at some point, learn to identify when a denial of coverage might be justified, given the evidence-based information at hand, and how, specifically, to explain this to patients and to formulate an alternate treatment plan.

5. *Residents should know how to partner with health care managers and health care providers to assess, coordinate, and improve health care and know how these activities can affect system performance.* Residents will need to understand how the patient perspective is an important element of "system perfor-

mance," in that the patients' perception of quality can drive the assessment, coordination, and improvement efforts in healthcare.

As in competency #3 listed above, residents are most likely to learn this competency by example. Those who have been successful at partnering with the healthcare providers in their own systems to achieve positive change must be identified and enlisted as educators in residency programs, particularly if they are physicians. Given the complexity of today's healthcare systems, especially at academic medical centers, the logistics of freeing up time for such individuals and perhaps providing direct or indirect compensation for teaching is no small matter, but if we are serious about these competencies, we will need to move beyond "take me back to the lecture hall" theoretical presentations to more practical, directly applicable educational content.

TWO SCENARIOS THAT REFLECT THE PATIENT PERSPECTIVE ON SYSTEMS-BASED PRACTICE

How would the current generation of patients understand what we are calling "systems-based practice"? While some patients may be familiar — if not conversant — with the healthcare system that serves them, the vast majority of patients will first become aware of the overarching "system" of healthcare over the issue of payment for medical services.

When coverage for treatment or services is denied, patients immediately see themselves as at odds with the system they have trusted to care for them. Regardless of how familiar or even comfortable they are with the idea that they are being cared for under a "systems-based" structure of healthcare, when they are denied coverage they are likely to seek the more traditional model of the patient-physician relationship — one in which the physician acts solely as a patient advocate and has no allegiance to a healthcare "system."

There is a range of possibilities with regards to how patients are likely to respond to the changes in healthcare delivery and the healthcare system as a whole, but it is helpful here to explore the patient perspective at two ends of the spectrum: one in which the patient primarily sees the physician in a positive light, despite having more negative views of the system as a whole, and one in which the physician is more closely identified as a part of the system, and thus, seen generally in a more negative light.

THE "SYMPATHETIC" PATIENT

In this scenario, patients see themselves as on the physician's side, in the sense that they realize how difficult it must be to practice with all the constraints of organized healthcare, with the added challenges of rapidly expanding medical knowledge and technology. In this perspective, patients are more likely to be understanding or forgiving of medical error, or more tolerant in terms of physicians' behavior or demeanor. Physicians sometimes invite or engender this approach by prefacing the discussion of difficult treatment decisions with statements like, "I know what I think is best, but they have my hands tied," or "I'll call and try to fight for you, but the final decision on coverage is theirs." Physicians are removing themselves from responsibility for the financial aspects of care and the implications of the decision, and attempting to preserve their role as primary patient advocate, while they work within a system that patients may see as treating them unfairly.

While two statements above lay out the conflict between individual healthcare professionals and the "system," the first statement more directly puts forth a potentially problematic assumption — namely, that what the physician thinks is best, is, indeed, the best treatment decision for that particular patient. This assumption is problematic because the physician's treatment decision may be based on his or her own training and practice experience, whereas the payer's denial of payment for the proposed treatment is likely to be based on more general, evidence-based clinical practice guidelines derived from a review of the medical literature. The second statement is less clear on physicians' claim to know what's best, but more strongly states the patient advocacy role that most patients expect from their physicians.

Residents should learn to recognize when a patient is speaking from the sympathetic perspective, and realize that they, as the physician "objects" of this sympathy, stand to gain, in that patients' kind and supportive words will often make their job easier. For patients, however, there may be a downside. Physicians who sense that patients are sympathetic to their conflicted relationship with the healthcare system may be more likely to forego the explanation and communication called for in the systems-based competencies. When sympathetic patients are asked to participate in assessment of their physicians' competency specifically, these patients may be less critical and discerning. They may become relatively passive in terms of advocating for themselves, or in identifying and confronting unprofessional physician behavior.

THE "ADVERSARIAL" PATIENT

Here, patients see their physician as having "sold out" to organized, for-profit, business-oriented medicine, and they may approach the physician/patient relationship with a basic mistrust and suspicion of the motives of the physician. In this perspective, patients see themselves as having to "fight" for their rights as patients, and, if they have the power to do so in the given healthcare system, the outcome may involve finding another physician. While some patients are already frustrated and angry before they even meet a physician, it is important to teach residents that they may unwittingly create "adversarial" patients by failing to address systems issues early in their relationships. Choosing not to make any comment or to ask any questions about systems issues may be interpreted by patients as complete and total agreement or compliance with what patients perceive as unfair treatment. It is interesting to note that this same lack of information or clarity may go unnoticed or unchallenged by patients with the "sympathetic" perspective. When asked to participate in assessing physician competency, patients with as adversarial perspective may be overly critical and negative in their evaluation of physician behavior. Likewise, relatively inexperienced physicians are likely to take the behavior of the adversarial patient personally, and, consequently, react negatively to these patients in all aspects of their relationships, not simply in communication and negotiation around the systems issues. Residents who see the adversarial behavior as a plea for better communication or more information, rather than a personal affront or insult, are likely to have more successful interactions with their patients, and perhaps somewhat less job-related stress.

FINDING MIDDLE GROUND

The above scenarios represent two extremes on a continuum in what admittedly is a multifaceted and complicated relationship, and residents will quickly learn that most patients will exhibit features of both attitudes at one time or another. Some patients may even approach their interactions with physicians with something like a "neutral" perspective, in which they are informed and aware of the constraints under which their physicians work, and perhaps have a healthy skepticism as to whether physicians will always "take their side," but are also reasonably confident that physicians have their best interests at heart, and will fight for their patients when the stakes are genuinely high. There is no doubt that physicians are less autonomous, in the traditional sense, in the current healthcare system, but they are far from powerless, especially when they have an understanding of the systems in which they practice. Residents who cultivate a working knowledge of the system as it pertains to their practice and as it affects the outcomes of their patients, and who develop the communication skills needed to convey this knowledge to patients when it is timely and relevant, are likely to have balanced, mutually beneficial relationships with both the patients they serve, and the systems in which they serve them.

CONCLUSION

Keeping the patient perspective in mind as we develop residency programs that meet the ACGME core competencies will ensure that the competencies achieve their primary goal — the overall improvement of medical care. Paying particular attention to the patient perspective as it applies to the "systems-based" competency is especially important, since so many patients and physicians say that the recent changes in healthcare towards systems-based care have compromised the patient-physician relationship.[4] Physicians need to identify themselves and their practice as "systems-based," since this is, in fact, what they are, and to learn ways to convey this to patients that show the positive aspects of the situation. Physicians can and will still be patient advocates, but they will need new skills and tools to do this in systems-based healthcare. The ACGME core competencies have the potential to provide these new skills, and its focus shows that it is doing so.

NOTES

1. C. Laine and F. Davidoff, "Patient-Centered Medicine: A Professional Revolution," *Journal of American Medical Association* 275 (1996): 152-6; W. Moore, "Medical Education: Speak to

Me before It's Too Late," *Health Services Journal* 107 (1997): 20-2.

2. Accreditation Council for Graduate Medical Education and American Board of Medical Specialties, "ACGME Outcome Project, 2002; *http:\\www.acgme..org\outcome* or see appendix 1.

3. R.M. Wachter et al., "Reorganizing an Academic Medical Service: Impact on Cost, Quality, Patient Satisfaction, and Education," *Journal of American Medical Association* 279 (1998): 1560-5.

4. M.G. Bloche, "Clinical Loyalties and the Social Purposes of Medicine," *Journal of American Medical Association* 281 (1999): 268-74.

13

Training Residents for Excellence in Systems-Based Clinical Practices: Management of Blood Draws in Critical Care Medicine as the Quintessential Outcome Measure

Evan G. DeRenzo, Phil Buescher, and Kirsten Alcorn

INTRODUCTION

In 1999, the Accreditation Council for Graduate Medical Education (ACGME) started its Outcome Project. Emerging out of concerns that residents were not being trained sufficiently to practice medicine in today's healthcare environment, by 2002 the Outcome Project had shaped six competency domains. These are:

1. Patient care,
2. Medical knowledge,
3. Practice-based learning and improvement,
4. Interpersonal and communication skills,
5. Professionalism, and
6. Systems-based practice.

The assumption grounding each of the six is the same; all six competencies echo the Aristotelian notion of the Golden Mean. That is, excellence in patient care comes from providing each patient with what that particular patient needs — not too much, not too little, but just the right amount and kinds of medical care at the right time in the right setting. Meeting this Aristotelian ideal and operationalizing the competence domains will require developing thinking in terms of systems and process, painting ancient images of the doctor-patient relationship into the pictures of twenty-first century medicine. No longer is the doctor-patient relationship envisioned in a vacuum. Competent contemporary medical practice will retain the best of the doctor-patient relationship while it appreciates that this core relationship is now situated at the center of a complex and far-flung healthcare system.

To begin shaping methods for evaluating the skills needed to practice sound medicine in today's healthcare environment, the Outcome Project is now developing assessment tools, work that is scheduled to be completed in 2006. To contribute to this effort, we suggest that training residents in the appropriate ordering and oversight of blood tests in the critical care setting is an ideal outcome measure to evaluate competence in systems-based clinical practice. Appropriate use of blood tests in the critical care setting is an inherently systems-based process that, additionally, integrates aspects of all six competency domains.

According to information on the ACGME website, educational assessment is intended to evaluate residents' attainment of competency-based objectives and to facilitate continuous improvement of the educational experience and resident and residency program performance.[1] The ACGME defines assessment "as the process of collecting, synthesizing, and interpreting information to aid decision making." These characteristics of the assessment process can be integrated into evaluating residents' test ordering behaviors and judgments in the critical care setting. Appropriateness in ordering blood tests is an ideal vehicle for assessment, as it is an inherently systems-based practice that integrates all six competency areas.

Central to patient care, obtaining blood tests involves a broad range of technical and business processes inside and outside a hospital. Additionally, it is a ubiquitous part of clinical care that is in need of quality improvement. Ordering blood tests is a core component of the care of critically ill patients that is presently poorly managed, with duplicate testing a well-identified clinical and resource management problem. Reducing unnecessary blood loss has implications for community health and the environment, as well as for improving patient care and hospital resource utilization.

That blood test ordering is highly measurable makes it an ideal outcome measure. Because enough residents rotate through a hospital's critical care/intensive care unit(s), such an outcome measure would provide a meaningful educational experience. Evaluating residents on the appropriateness of their requests for blood tests in a critical care unit marries all six competencies, exemplifying especially how competence in patient care practices translates into excellence in internal process management and vice versa: that excellence in systems-based practice contributes to excellence in clinical care. An Outcome Project outcome measure that could serve the dual purpose of providing measurable evaluation of residents and residency programs performance and concurrently elevating the quality of blood draw practices within the critical care units of a hospital would be a valuable outcome measure indeed.

WHY TRAINING RESIDENTS IN APPROPRIATE BLOOD DRAW PRACTICES IN CRITICAL CARE IS NEEDED

The need to reduce unnecessary blood tests in hospitalized, critically ill patients has been recognized for decades. Although anemia in hospitalized patients, particularly the critically ill, is multifactorial, recognition of iatrogenic anemia in hospitalized patients is well-established.[2] Data demonstrate higher incidence of iatrogenic anemia and transfusion requirements in the critically ill, especially in intensive and/or coronary care unit patients in whom blood draws are the most frequent in the hospital.[3] Although the relevance of iatrogenic anemia and transfusion to gross patient outcomes is unclear[4] and controversy continues around what the best hematocrit trigger for transfusion should be,[5] clinical judgment is strong that harms such as stress on cardiovascular and respiratory systems and exposure to bloodborne pathogens are reduced by minimization of blood loss and less frequent transfusions.[6]

The literature includes several additional reasons pointing to the need for improvement in blood test ordering practices. First among these is protecting colleagues and coworkers from sharps injuries. The incidence of needlestick injuries in the

United States is estimated to be roughly 4 percent per 10,000, although the actual numbers are expected to be higher than that reported.[7] The potential for infecting healthcare workers with HIV and hepatitis B and C is an occupational hazard of immeasurable ethical, medical, and fiscal concern. Even when needlestick injuries do not result in infection transmission, the psychological distress produced by the injury can be severe. These psychological harms include fear, anxiety, and emotional distress, and will sometimes be pronounced enough to result in occupational and behavior changes. One study attempting to examine these less-tangible harms found that the subjects, all of whom had recently experienced a sharps injury, would have been willing to pay substantial out-of-pocket costs to have had a sharps-injury prevention program at their hospital to avoid the emotional distress the injury had caused them.[8] Preventing physical and mental harm to healthcare workers is as strong a moral obligation as is the moral obligation to protect patients, and is a key component to professionalism within a systems context.

Concerns about the impact of unnecessary blood tests extend beyond the hospital's critically ill patients and staff. Accountability to the community from which a hospital's patients come is another system requiring attention and consideration. Concern for a hospital's effect on the well-being of the community in which the facility is geographically situated is an important organizational ethics consideration and is integral to demonstrating physician professionalism within a systems-based practice. That is, because blood is a scarce resource, when patients come into a hospital needing blood, it is important that the hospital's blood stores have not been depleted avoidably. Drawing down on these resources inappropriately puts the hospital's community population at risk. When a hospital's blood bank is depleted by patients who need transfusions because they have lost blood needlessly, the potential harms are more than doubled. Under these conditions, blood resources have been given to patients who could have avoided the risks that blood transfusion poses, while those who need blood transfusion out of legitimate emergency medical need do not have blood available to them. There is no predicting when a hospital could be inundated with emergencies that stretch its blood bank to the maximum. Efficient utilization of this scarce resource is a professional obligation of both physicians and hospitals, to both patients and the community.

Management of blood waste is both a business concern for hospitals as well as an environmental concern for hospitals' immediate and broader communities, and this is another organizational ethics issue to which physicians should be attentive. Today, concerns about medical waste have become a global issue.[9] Under the United Kingdom and Wales's Environmental Protection Act of 1990, hospitals have what is referred to as a "duty to care" to assure that disposal of hospital waste does not cause harm to human health or the environment.[10] These concerns are sometimes referred to as "greening" the environment, that is, being environmentally responsible. In the hospital context, greening is spoken of as "collective interdisciplinary organizational behavior that reduces environmental hazards and overconsumption."[11] In the U.S., a group has formed called Hospitals for a Healthy Environment (H2E). It is a national program designed to assist hospitals across the country to improve their waste-disposal practices. Clearly improvement is needed. In the U.S., hospitals have become serious polluters, using 10 percent of all energy used and producing thousands of tons of waste daily.[12] In short, hospitals and their personnel ought to act as good citizens with respect to the physical environment. One obvious way to do this is to produce less waste by reducing overconsumption through reducing unnecessary blood tests.

Various approaches to reducing unnecessary blood test ordering have been considered and/or implemented such as special awareness education programs[13] and practice guidelines,[14] using pediatric tubes for pediatric patients and adults, making technological changes in instrumentation and waste management strategies, and instituting hospital blood conservation committees[15] or other administratively implemented policies and procedures.[16] Progress, however, has been slow. Further, these efforts have lacked the force necessary to produce meaningful, systemwide change. Turning appropriate blood draw practices in the critical care setting into an outcomes measure for resident training could be the new, targeted strategy that is needed to serve as a "tipping point"[17] in producing sustainable reductions in wasteful blood draw practices and in advancing resident education. Using critical care blood testing behavior as an outcome measure promises to train the next generation of physicians to avoid blood wastage, and, in so doing, creates the likelihood that the many harms that unnecessary blood loss can produce may ultimately be eliminated from the healthcare system.

WHY BLOOD TEST ORDERING IN CRITICAL CARE IS AN IDEAL OUTCOME MEASURE FOR THE ACGME COMPETENCY IN SYSTEMS-BASED PRACTICE

Competency in systems-based practice requires that residents "demonstrate an awareness of and responsiveness to the larger context and system of healthcare and the ability to effectively call on system resources to provide care that is of optimal value." Appropriate ordering of blood tests demonstrates all that is called for in this competency, and it integrates demonstration of additional competencies. For example, efficient resource management and the practice of cost-effective healthcare are demonstrated by appreciating the relationship of optimal blood test ordering in the critically ill to the management of blood bank resources. Residents could be encouraged to participate in a blood conservation program planning process, which would teach them the difference between inappropriate blood rationing at the bedside and appropriate policy-level considerations that establish fair triggers for review limits on transfusions, a competency requirement for professionalism.[18] That is, residents caring for critically ill patients at the end of life with end-stage disease, who also require blood, may intuitively make the choice not to advocate for additional transfusions on the basis that the patient is dying anyway so giving the blood to this patient wastes blood another patient may need. Participating in a hospital blood conservation program, however, can teach residents invaluable ethical lessons about the difference between having hospital policies that elevate the approval of blood unit use to another physician or to a transfusion committee, so that the primacy of the physician's obligations for the care and advocacy for the patient is not degraded by inappropriate considerations for others at the bedside.

Additionally, knowing when or when not to order a blood test also involves practice-based learning about ethical norms that are related, more broadly, to optimal end-of-life care. Residents demonstrate professionalism when they integrate judgments about blood test ordering in the critically ill when shifting from aggressive life-extending technologies to comfort care — when blood tests for diagnostic purposes may best be withheld.

Another example of integrating competency in systems-based practice with competencies in patient care and professionalism relates to residents who care for persons who are practicing Jehovah's Witnesses. Competency in professionalism requires that residents demonstrate sensitivity and responsiveness to patients' culture, which includes religious belief. The case of a critically ill Jehovah's Witness patient presents the resident with an important opportunity to care for a patient in a way that advances the resident's attention to blood conservation and the scientific data on managing patients who refuse blood products.[19] Because the technology of blood product substitution has advanced markedly over the last several decades, many hospitals have initiated bloodless programs to meet the clinical needs of Jehovah's Witness patients. Where such programs exist, they can be excellent teaching tools for residents about technological progress in this area. Where hospitals do not have such programs, residents will need to advance their own learning, demonstrating additional competencies such as investigating medical knowledge and supporting their own education, to assure they demonstrate competency in professionalism.

Yet another aspect of competency in systems-based practice, which can be demonstrated by appropriate ordering of blood tests, is social accountability for protecting the community and the environment. Systems-based competency calls for residents to demonstrate an understanding of how their patient care practices affect others in society, at large. As already noted, social accountability is demonstrated by judicious blood bank resource management. Residents are accountable to the global community when sound healthcare practices reduce healthcare costs, generally, and reduce the amounts and kinds of medical waste released into the environment. Professionalism in accountability to one's colleagues and the profession is demonstrated by reducing behaviors that put colleagues at unnecessary risk of sharps injuries.

Competency in systems-based practice calls for residents to practice cost-effective healthcare and to utilize resources so as not to compromise the quality of care. Attention to efficient resource management is addressed by virtually all aspects of reducing unnecessary blood draws in critically ill patients. Cost savings for reduced numbers of sharps injuries could be substantial.[20] Laboratory costs, estimated to be approximately 6 percent of the total costs for surgical conditions and 9 percent of the total costs for medical conditions, could be reduced.[21] Reducing the need for transfusions could save money in laboratory expenditures and patient care.[22] Appropriate blood test ordering provides critically ill patients with care that is of optimal value by reducing the possibility that they will develop iatrogenic anemia or require blood transfusions that might otherwise have been avoided, addressing the patient care competency's requirement to provide healthcare services aimed at preventing health problems.

Competency in patient care also requires that residents provide care that is compassionate, appropriate, and effective. Included in this competency domain are the abilities to gather essential information, to make informed decisions about diagnosis, and to use information technology to support patient care decisions. Blood testing, as a primary route to excellence in diagnosis and patient care management, demands skill in these abilities. Even in those hospitals that have practice guidelines and/or pre-designated order sets that are designed to provide consistency and guidance in blood test ordering, such practice aides ought not to be used without considering the appropriateness to each patient's clinical status. Overriding such guidelines is sometimes required for optimal patient care.

Systems-based practice competency requires residents to know how various delivery systems differ. By only having necessary blood tests, patients will not have their insurance companies charged for unnecessary tests and the hospital will not be responsible for unnecessary care that is uncompensated. This competency domain requires, also, that residents demonstrate an ability to advocate for quality patient care and to assist patients in navigating system complexities. Few things are more complicated from a systems perspective than the problem of duplicate orders for blood tests. Especially in critically ill patients who have easy blood draw access, blood conservation is particularly challenging. Critically ill patients are often seen by a number of subspecialty consultants, and it is well-known that duplicated tests, ordered by multiple physicians, are a serious source of unnecessary blood loss.[23] House staff could be evaluated on the degree to which they did not order a test that was requested by a consultant that was duplicative, or on the thoroughness with which residents read specialist's notes, in which duplicated orders may be embedded. Hospital laboratory reports that identify and/or cancel duplicated orders within set time frames could be used to validate this sort of assessment, and the degree to which residents utilize such hospital systems could demonstrate competency in practice-based learning. Additionally, the degree to which residents effectively communicate with their peers and with other professionals, both above and below them on the medical hierarchy, about reversing an order for a duplicated blood test will demonstrate how skilled residents are at advocating for the well-being of their patients and in assisting their patients in navigating system complexities. Such evaluation addresses competencies in systems-based practice, as well as requirements in the competency on interpersonal and communication skills to demonstrate effective information exchange and on teaming with professional associates. While knowing when not to order or re-order a blood test in a critically ill patient is one aspect of cost-effective quality healthcare, as required by skilled systems-based practice, it is also a demonstration of expertise in medical knowledge. Assessing residents' medical knowledge in the area of the utility of blood tests will help residency program supervisors determine if residents know and apply basic and clinical research data to their blood test ordering practices.

Differentiating between tests ordered on the basis of evidence-based medicine, rather than as the result of uncritical thinking about routinized practice, can yield valid data about residents' scientific knowledge. For example, residents could be tested on whether or not they know that the majority of critically ill patients are anemic at admission to the intensive care units (ICUs), that hemoglobin concentrations typically decline during the first three days of the ICU stay,[24] and that, although transfusion may be beneficial in life-threatening anemia, there are mounting data regarding adverse clinical outcomes for transfusion in the critically ill.[25] The same might apply to determining if residents were developing bad habits, such as ordering blood tests on critically ill patients who have indwelling catheters for fever work-ups that require substantial amounts of blood that may provide little useful information.[26] This kind of information could be of use to residency programs in identifying areas of medical knowledge that can influence residents' test ordering judgments and patterns and that, therefore, need to be well covered during resident training lectures.

CONCLUSION

Shaping appropriate blood test ordering in critically ill patients is an ideal outcome measure for several reasons. Test ordering is measurable. Resident supervisors can evaluate whether or not tests ordered were appropriate. Thorough review of the chart should provide evidence of whether or not duplicate tests were ordered and/or obtained. Knowing when and when not to order a blood test in a critically ill patient is central to a maturing physician's ability to provide excellent clinical care. Excellence in clinical care integrates all six ACGME competency domains, and is essentially a systems-based practice. Systems-based practice requires that residents demonstrate an awareness of and responsiveness to the larger context and systems in which they practice. Residents must learn to effectively and efficiently utilize systems resources to the benefit of their patients. Residents who demonstrate systems-based competence in blood test ordering patterns in the critically ill can be expected to understand how their practice of medicine affects other patients, professionals, and healthcare systems. Sharpened skills in ordering blood tests and reducing duplication by others in critical care will teach residents to be cost-effective clinicians who do not compromise the quality of patient care. By focusing on blood draw outcomes, residents will learn how to effectively partner with other players and sectors of the healthcare system to achieve optimal patient care outcomes.

That is why taking the matter of blood drawing in the critically ill and shaping it into a competency outcomes assessment measure fits neatly into the goals of the Outcome Project. Test ordering practices are habituated early in a resident's program. Residents learn test ordering habits from the models of the senior residents, the resident training supervisors, the attendings, and the consultants with whom they interact. Making critical care test ordering appropriateness a competency outcome measure will establish the importance of precision in this systems-influencing practice early in the resident's medical career. To be successful at systems-based practice related to efficient use of blood tests requires integration of all the competencies to navigate the multiple layers of a hospital's many functions and departments. Working to actively reduce the numbers of unnecessary blood tests that one's critically ill patients receive can teach residents about how their patient care practices affect others throughout the hospital. Learning to pay particular attention to reducing blood waste contributes to enhanced patient care, protects the scarce resource of banked blood, and helps to control hospital, health insurance, and waste management costs — when less money is spent by the hospital on unnecessary tests, there may be an increased ability to pay for necessary but uncompensated care. In sum, the many benefits can have positive ripple effects throughout all of the systems that make up our complex, modern healthcare system.

DISCLAIMER

The opinions expressed in this chapter are those of the authors' only and do not represent any positions or policies of any organization to which any of the authors are affiliated.

NOTES

1. *http://www.acgme.org/acWebsite/home/home.asp.*
2. E. Eyster and J. Bernene, "Nosocomial Anemia," *Journal of the American Medical Association* 223 (1973): 73-4; E. Gleason et al., "Minimizing Diagnostic Blood Loss in Critically Ill Patients," *American Journal of Critical Care* 1 (1992): 85-90; J.C. Dale and S. G. Ruby, "Specimen Collection Volumes for Laboratory Tests: A College of American Pathologists Study of 140 Laboratories," *Archives of Pathology and Laboratory Medicine* 127 (2003):162-68.
3. Z. F. Dech and N. L. Szaflarski, "Nursing Strategies to Minimize Blood Loss Associated with Phlebotomy," *AACN Clinical Issues: Advanced Practice in Acute and Critical Care* 7, no. 2 (1996): 277-287; K. U. Eckardt, "Anemia in Critical Illness," *Wien Klin Wochenschr.* 113, no. 3-4 (2001): 84-89; D. Wisser et al., "Blood Loss From Laboratory Tests," *Clinical Chemistry* 49, no. 10 (2001): 1651-5; P. Carroll, "Blood Conservation Strategies in Cardiovascular Surgery," *Dimensions of Critical Care Nursing* 24, no. 3 (2005): 152.
4. C. M. MacIsaac et al., "The Influence of a Blood Conserving Device on Anemia in Intensive Care Patients," *Anaesthesia and Intensive Care* 31, no. 6 (2003): 653-7; D. Wisser et al., see note 3 above; A. Shander, "Anemia in the Critically Ill," *Critical Care Nursing Clinics* 20, no. 2 (2004): 159-78.
5. M. I. Rudis et al., "Managing Anemia in the Critically Ill Patient," *Pharmacotherapy* 24, no. 2 (2004): 229-47.
6. R. A. Fowler et al., "Blood Conservation for Critically Ill

Patients," *Critical Care Nursing Clinics* 20, no. 2 (2004): 313-24; H. L. Corwin, "Transfusion Practice in the Critically Ill: Can We Do Better?" *Critical Care Medicine* 33, no. 1 (2005): 232-3.

7. J. C. Trim and T. S. Elliott, "A Review of Sharps Injuries and Preventative Strategies," *Journal of Hospital Infection* 53, no. 4 (2003): 237-42; A. L. Panlilio et al., "Estimate of the Annual Number of Percutaneous Injuries among Hospital-Based Healthcare Workers in the United States, 1997-1998," *Infection Control and Hospital Epidemiology* 25 (2004): 556-562; J. M. Lee et al., "Needlestick Injuries in the United States: Epidemiologic, Economic, and Quality of Life Issues," *AAOHN Journal* 53, no. 3 (2005): 117-33.

8. D. N. Fisman et al., "Willingness to Pay to Avoid Sharps-Related Injuries: A Study in Injured Health Care Workers," *American Journal of Infection Control* 30, no. 5 (2002): 283-7.

9. C. Wichmann et al., "Inflammatory Activity in River-Water Samples," *Environmental Toxicology and Chemistry* 19 (2004): 594-602; F. Uysal and E. Tinmaz, "Medical Waste Management in Trachea Region of Turkey: Suggested Remedial Action," *Waste Management Research Report* 22, no. 5 (2004): 403-7; M. Burd, "Reducing the Risks Related to the Handling and Disposal of Health-Care Waste," *Professional Nurse* 20, no. 8 (2005): 40-2; A. V. Sergeev and D. O. Carpenter, "Hospitalization Rates for Coronary Heart Disease in Relation to Residence Near Areas Contaminated with Persistent Organic Pollutants and other Pollutants," *Environmental Health Perspectives* 113, no. 6 (2005): 756-61; N. Marinkovic et al., "Hazardous Medical Waste Management as a Public Health Issue," *Arh Hig Rada Toksikol* 56, no. 1 (2005): 21-32.

10. P. Tearle, "Clinical Waste Management," *Communicable Disease and Public Health* 4, no. 3 (2001): 234-236.

11. M. Topft, "Psychological Explanations and Interventions for Indifference to Greening Hospitals," *Health Care Management Review* 30, no. 1 (2005): 2-8.

12. L. Brannen, "Managing Medical Waste," *Health Progress* 84, no. 6 (November-December 2003):25-28.

13. Trim and Elliott, see note 7 above; D. Beland, C. D'Angelo, and D. Vinci, "Reducing unnecessary blood work in the neurological ICU," *Journal of Neuroscience Nursing* 35, no. 30 (2003): 149-52.

14. T.J. Wang et al., "A utilization management intervention

to reduce unnecessary testing in the coronary care unit," *Archives of Internal Medicine* 162, no. 16 (2002): 1885-90.

15. W.H. Dzik et al., "Patient safety and blood transfusion: new solutions," *Transfusion Medicine Reviews* 17, no. 3 (2003): 169-80; S.L. Haynes and F. Torella, "The role of hospital transfusion committees in blood product conservation," *Transfusion Medicine Reviews* 18, no. 2 (2004): 93-104.

16. K. Lewandrowski, "Managing utilization of new diagnostic tests," *Clinical Leadership Management Review* 17, no. 6 (2003): 318-24; M.D. McNeely, "The use of ordering protocols and other maneuvers: the Canadian experience," *Clinical Laboratory Medicine* 22, no. 2 (2002): 505-14.

17. M. Gladwell, *The Tipping Point: How Little Things Can Make a Big Difference* (New York: Little, Brown, 2000).

18. J.P. Aubuchon, L. Petz, and A. Fink, *Policy Alternatives in Transfusion Medicine* (Bethesda, Md.: AABB Press, 2001).

19. Z.M. Bodnaruk, C.J. Wong, and M.J. Thomas, "Meeting the clinical challenge of care for Jehovah's Witnesses," *Transfusion Medicine Reviews* 18, no. 2 (2004): 105-16.

20. F. Roudot-Thoraval et al., "Costs and benefits of measures to prevent needlestick injuries in a university hospital," *Infection Control & Hospital Epidemiology* 20 (1999): 614-7.

21. D.S. Young, B.S. Sachais, and L.C. Jefferies, "Laboratory Costs in the Context of Disease," *Clinical Chemistry* 46, no. 7 (2000): 967-75; B. Custer, "Economic analyses of blood safety and transfusion medicine interventions: a systematic review," *Transfusion Medicine Reviews* 18, no. 2 (2004): 127-43.

22. B.D. Spiess, "Blood conservation: Why bother?" *Journal of Cardiothoracic and Vascular Anesthesia* 18, no. 4 (August 2004 supp.): 1S-5S.

23. P. Valenstein, A. Leiken, C. Lehmann, "Test-ordering by multiple physicians increases unnecessary laboratory examinations," *Archives of Pathology and Laboratory Medicine* 112 (1988): 238-41; B.R. Smoller, M.S. Kruskall, and G.L. Horowitz, "Reducing adult phlebotomy blood loss with the use of pediatric-sized blood collection tubes," *American Journal of Clinical Pathology* 91, no. 6 (1989): 701-3; P. Valenstein and R.B. Schifman, "Duplicate laboratory orders: A College of American Pathologists Q-Probes Study of Thyrotropin Requests in 502 Institutions," *Archives of Pathology and Laboratory Medicine* 120, no. 10 (1996): 917-21; E.G. Neilson et al., "The impact of peer management on

test-ordering behavior," report for the Resource Utilization Committee, *Annals of Internal Medicine* 141, no. 3 (2004): 196-204.

24. Fowler, see note 6 above.

25. Shander, see note 4 above; B.D. Spiess, "Risks of transfusion: outcome focus," *Transfusion* 44, supp. (2004): 4S-14S.

26. P.S. Barie, "Phlebotomy in the intensive care unit: strategies for blood conservation," *Critical Care* 8, supp. 2 (2004): S34-6.

Summary and Conclusion

*Ann E. Mills, Donna T. Chen,
Patricia H. Werhane, and Matthew K. Wynia*

Academic health centers are scrambling to implement the ACGME competencies, including the two competencies we have focused on throughout this book: the competency on professionalism and the competency on systems-based practice. The fact that the competency on professionalism includes a requirement that residents should commit to the ethical principles associated with business practices has been largely, if not completely, overlooked until recently.[1] Not only does this requirement have profound implications for medical professionalism as physicians traditionally understand it, it directly links medical professionalism to systems-based practice.

"Professionalism" means different things to different people and to different groups of people. In the context of healthcare, different organizations, like the American Medical Association (AMA) and the various professional bodies to which physicians of different specialties belong, emphasize different components of it. But the component of medical professionalism that society has most strongly endorsed, that society understands, that society wants to believe in, is the component that requires physicians to put personal interests aside and to act as patient advocates. This is why, as a society, we are so dismayed when physicians, for whatever reason, act or make decisions that actually — or seem to — undermine or ignore patients' best interests.

The ACGME competency on professionalism also includes a different commitment — a commitment to the ethical principles of business practices — and this commitment has the potential to undermine medical professionalism as we have traditionally understood it. This is because it is perceived, rightly or wrongly, that "business practices" generally reflect a commitment to cost savings or cost-effectiveness. We have seen in the managed-care revolution how uneasily the two related values, quality and cost-effectiveness, co-mingle in the context of healthcare.[2] But the ACGME has also offered a way out of this conundrum — it has added to the competency on systems-based practice a requirement that physicians understand the systems in which they work, be able to differentiate between them, and work to improve them.[3]

As the authors in this book have described, there are difficulties with this approach. There are conceptual difficulties associated with the organizational and macro systems in which physicians work and physicians' relationships to these systems. In addition, there are problems that arise from the traditional perspectives of physicians. We will summarize the insights offered by the authors of this book below.

• • •

All systems reflect the values associated with their goals. For instance, a system designed to be cost-effective will reflect the values of cost-effectiveness. Systems designed to produce outcomes that meet the expectations of customers will value "customer satisfaction." Because the goals and the values associated with these two types of systems are different, we can expect them to exhibit different characteristics. For instance, systems associated with cost-effectiveness might be rigid, while systems associated with customer satisfaction might be more flexible.[4]

Different systems may interact with one another, and the different values that are reflected in them might be appropriate, or not, depending on context.[5] For instance, a diner might experience customer satisfaction if his or her meal was prepared and served appropriately, which might mean wait staff having the ability to react to the diner's wishes with a large degree of flexibility. Even so, the diner expects the bill to be rigorously prepared. Flexibility in the systems that prepare the bill will not be tolerated by the diner.

Summary and Conclusion 255

In the healthcare context, systems are seen in the micro context, as in a physician practice. They are also seen in a mid-level or macro context, as the organization with which the physician interacts or the delivery system as a whole. It is generally the case that once the physician or the patient moves from one-on-one individual encounters, they will both be embedded in one or more different systems. Difficulties arise when the goals and values of a particular individual, organization, or system are inappropriate for the context, as for instance, when patient and physician have different expectations arising out of their encounter, or when patient care procedures reflect cost concerns at the expense of quality care, or when two or more systems reflect different values, so that they interact inappropriately as, for instance, in the case discussed in the chapter "Educating for Systems-Informed Professionalism." In these situations confusion within the system is inevitable and inappropriate results are probable. And because, in the healthcare context, as in any service industry, systems are composed of persons interacting together to produce the goal of the system, there will likely be unhappiness and dissatisfaction by the people working in it — with its design, the interactions it produces, and the outcomes it is producing.

Inconsistent and inappropriate values in the systems that make up our healthcare delivery system produce inconsistent and inappropriate outcomes.[6] Physicians,[7] as well as patients and their families, are unhappy with the U.S. healthcare system as it is currently constructed and they are showing dissatisfaction with the mid level system — the healthcare organization.[8] But physicians, at least individually, do not have the power to affect or influence these larger systems. Often they have limited power to affect the systems that make up the organizations with which they interact. So one conceptual difficulty in terms of the ACGME competencies is this: How can physicians commit to the ethical principles of business practices when, in macro and mid level contexts, like the whole of delivery system or in healthcare organizations, they often have little or no control over them?

The traditional perspective of the physician has been to isolate the patient-physician encounter from the systems that surround both the patient and the physician and to see this encounter as the beginning and end of the physician's professional responsibility. To be sure, this perspective has changed somewhat, as physicians have understood the implications of the managed-care revolution — and the encroachment on their ability to make medical decisions. Nevertheless, the individual encounter remains the dominant mental model with which physicians view and evaluate their professionalism. The competencies, however, have called for a wider perspective, one that is capable of understanding and evaluating system performance. Thus, new knowledge, skills, and sensitivities are required.

A systems perspective must take into account the elements or components of a system which, as we have said, are its purpose, processes, necessary resources, and effectiveness. Each of these elements corresponds to an area identified by Robert S. Kaplan and David P. Norton in the Balanced Scorecard framework they developed.[9] Donna Chen, Ann Mills, and Patricia Werhane used that framework to develop what they call a "systems-informed perspective," which may in itself help structure the requirements of competency in systems-based practice. But while a systems-informed perspective might help in understanding systems and identifying areas for improvement, it cannot guide decision making directly. This requires setting out goals and values, and prioritizing them. Because we are dealing with healthcare, these goals and values are found in the goals and values that are associated with medical professionalism, which reflect the values endorsed by society as being appropriate for healthcare, and that now, according to the ACGME, should also include consideration of the ethical principles associated with business practices. The incorporation of medical professionalism and the values associated with it can move us from a "systems-informed perspective" towards "systems-informed *professionalism.*"

Chen, Mills, and Werhane do not suggest that systems-informed professionalism will put an end to all conflict within the systems that surround the delivery of care. There are two reasons for this. First, men and women of integrity and intelligence can and will disagree on appropriate solutions to systems problems. More importantly, this model is designed to be used primarily in an organizational context (although it can be used at both the micro and the more macro level of the delivery system). For systems-informed professionalism to have any practical effect, the organizational culture, of which the ethical climate is an important part, must support its use. [10] This means the ethical climate must support and encourage the values associated with the medical profession. This brings us a potential solution to the problems that are inherent in the ACGME approach to reconfiguring the expertise that future physicians must have.

THE ROLE OF ORGANIZATIONAL ETHICS FOR SYSTEMS-INFORMED PROFESSIONALISM

As we outlined in the introduction to this volume, one of the aims of organizational ethics for healthcare is to create and sustain a positive ethical climate in the healthcare organization.[11] Thus organizational ethics is necessarily concerned with what affects the ethical climate, and, in healthcare organizations, this includes the systems surrounding the delivery of care. We have identified the characteristics of a system as having four elements: purpose, process, resources, and effectiveness. Therefore, if organizational ethics is concerned with systems of care, it is concerned with the characteristics of the systems employed by the organization to deliver care.

Organizational ethics focuses on the purpose or the mission of the healthcare organization, and whether or not the systems that support the organization's functioning reflect its declared mission, goals, and values. One might argue that systems always reflect an organization's true goals and values, but that these are often left unstated — hence, one goal for organizational ethics is to reconcile an organization's stated goals with the goals its systems of care are designed to promote. This means organizational ethics is, or should be, concerned with whether or not these systems are designed in ways that reflect the organization's stated goals and values. If organizational ethics is concerned with the design of systems, it is also concerned with the use of resources and with the human beings who interact in these systems. Finally, one of the activities of organizational ethics is to evaluate whether or not a particular system is effective and financially viable, because these issues will affect how resources are used. All of these components interact to inform the individuals working within the organization of the values of their specific organization. These characteristics will likely affect the beliefs and behaviors of individuals interacting together in a healthcare organization, and, as discussed earlier, *this* creates the ethical climate of the healthcare organization. By analogy, on a macro level, how healthcare organizations interact with larger systems affects the organization, its ethical climate, and its values.

How does a positive ethical climate help in the resolution of the problems associated with requiring physicians working in complex healthcare systems to commit to professionalism, which includes a commitment to ethical principles associated with business practices? First, how does a positive ethical climate allow physicians to retain their traditional sense of professionalism while simultaneously making a commitment to the ethical principles associated with business practices? The answer is that it does so by ensuring that the business practices or systems with which physicians interact reflect the values associated with professionalism. In this way, physicians should not experience a conflict between their own sense of professionalism and the systems with which they interact. Is this possible? Is it realistic? We believe so.

It is certainly possible for healthcare organizations involved in residency training to create, as Evan DeRenzo suggests, a "morally safe environment" for their residents. DeRenzo describes vignettes that illustrate how the environment affects the beliefs and behaviors of those interacting with residents. Her stories illustrate how difficult change would be. David Ozar makes a similar point. This is not surprising. Changes in beliefs and behaviors in any organization are often difficult, and, more often than not, they take a long time — possibly years.[12] But healthcare organizations that are involved in residency training have the power to affect change internally, and they have the responsibility to change if they are to meet the requirements of the ACGME competencies. Looking to organizations and their ethical climates puts the responsibility for change where it should be — in the organization — while simultaneously allowing individual residents to investigate the possibility of change without fear of being penalized. But what about the environment external to the organization — the larger macro set of systems with which it interacts? Throughout this book, various authors have contended that residents and other physicians have little or no power to change the external environment (except through professional associations and organizations). But healthcare organizations do, to some extent, have this power.

While at times it may not seem the case, healthcare organizations and the leaders associated with them can affect the larger

Summary and Conclusion

environment (that is, the delivery system as a whole) and thus can help ensure that systems reflect appropriate values. Healthcare organizations interact with and in the external environment. They negotiate with payers, both private and governmental. And if, individually (like physicians), they are sometimes at a disadvantage in these negotiations, they are members of associations like the American Hospital Association (AHA) and the Association of American Medical Colleges. Their interventions in the larger delivery system have often been successful, especially when they work together with physician organizations. For instance, currently the AHA is engaged, with other like-minded organizations, including the AMA, in the controversy over medical liability.[13] Whether or not one agrees with the solutions these organizations have proposed, working together they *have* had some success. Legislative reforms are inching their way through the House and Senate,[14] and some states have passed reform measures capping awards for non-economic damages and structuring annuities instead of large payouts for future care.[15] Furthermore, the healthcare delivery system, as the Institute of Medicine has pointed out, is a complex adaptive system, and thus has the power to affect change through its interactions with larger political and other social systems.[16] These interactions will determine whether we can move incrementally to the development of a systems ethic that incorporates, as Edward Spencer and Rebecca Bigoney note, the traditional values associated with healthcare delivery.

It may seem that we are implying that change is easy. It is not. For one thing, healthcare organizations must be concerned with the competitive landscape they face. Sometimes positive change is rewarded, but sometimes change by only one player, without change in the underlying system, can be punished in the marketplace. For instance, there is at present only a very weak, or no, business case for improving quality of care when doing so does not save money.[17] As this is the case, if healthcare organizations are interested in delivering high quality care, then all healthcare organizations, along with physicians, must commit to the values associated with professionalism, and, importantly, advocate for these values within larger social systems.[18]

We also do not mean to imply that conflict will not occur. It will — even among organizations that share the same values. Competition in the healthcare market is intense and is likely to remain so, and dollar margins in most healthcare organizations are slim. Achieving a systems ethic would be easier, however, if healthcare organizations and other mid level organizational systems that make up the macro healthcare delivery system could agree on the values this larger system should reflect, and on how these values should be prioritized — *and evidence the will to change*. Although it will not be easy, we believe this is possible.[19]

Furthermore, the ACGME competencies have called for a change in the perspective of future physicians; a positive ethical climate is required for that as well. Chen, Mills, and Werhane have developed a perspective they call systems-informed professionalism. The mental model it encourages can be useful in fulfilling the ACGME competencies. But the model also relies on decision making being guided by professional values, which now include both traditional professional values and the ethical principles associated with business practices. If these values are not respected, encouraged, and reflected in the ethical climates of organizations and macro systems, ethical climate, then, as a practical matter, this perspective will be useless, as the decisions it points to cannot be made by the responsible individual.

• • •

We have divided this book into sections that correspond to the components of the Balanced Scorecard framework. We have asked various scholars, administrators, and practicing physicians to give us insights into each component. In addition, we have asked authors to consider how and what to teach residents.

Nevertheless, the problems we have discussed above remain. We have identified and discussed some potential solutions to these problems, most of which rely on organizational and professional commitments to the ethics of healthcare at all levels. But we are obliged to admit that organizational ethics programs or the persons who are charged with the development and enhancement of a positive ethical climate are today the exception, not the rule, in healthcare organizations. There are reasons for this, including a lack of time and money, the possibility of duplicate functions, et cetera. Yet one of the more serious problems, as we see it, is lack of interest due to an ingrained belief that we as physicians *do act* professionally — and that persons associated with healthcare organizations already know the values that are associated with healthcare and act on them. Thus, the assumption is that worrying about the ethical climate of healthcare organizations is superfluous, not important to professional decision making, and that healthcare organizations need no help in encouraging the integration of these values in day-to-day activities. Becker and Goodman's essay describes some of the enormous frustrations and tensions that doctors are under and they offer "mindfulness" both as a way to alleviate that stress and to strive for reflective practice. To be sure, some frustrations and tensions will arise simply because of the nature of clinical work, but Daniel Becker and Matthew Goodman seem less concerned with stress arising from these activities and more concerned with the awkward positions in which physicians sometimes find themselves because of the constraints and characteristics of the systems with which and in which they work. From the physician's perspective, this ethical tension (some have called it "moral distress"[20]) arises from the fact that the values of patient care, to which they are committed as their most important concern, are not universally shared by the macro environments in which they must practice — which include healthcare organizations and the healthcare system as a whole. This distress is evident throughout the essays in this book.

Real change is necessary if the ACGME is correct that the evolving healthcare system requires future physicians to master the areas of expertise they have outlined, and, hence, that residency training programs must produce graduates that evidence real competence in the knowledge, skills, and sensitivities they specify. Otherwise, the introduction of the new competencies will be an additional burden that residents and the academic health centers with which they are associated will simply pretend to acquire to be accredited. If this happens, we might have to add this initiative to the long list of failures we have seen as our society attempts to discover ways to deliver high quality, cost-effective care. On the other hand, if real change is encouraged, if academic health centers take the lead, as they must, if they are sincere about fulfilling the requirements of the ACGME competencies, we might begin to see the development of a systems ethic that can be agreed upon by all components of the delivery system. Such a change is much needed, and it is our hope that the work of the ACGME in showing how professional ethics must guide the healthcare system — and how physicians and the organizations in which they work can help shape the healthcare system — will prove to be the starting point.

NOTES

1. On 6 September 2005, we did a searched Medline on the words "ACGME" "competencies." We drew 74 essays. We then added the terms "business practices" and/or "business ethics" and drew zero results.

2. J.C. Robinson, "The End of Managed Care," *Journal of American Medical Association* 285, no. 20 (May 2001): 2622-8. Also see J.D. Kleinke. *Bleeding Edge — The Business of Health Care in the New Century* (Gaithersburg, Md.: Aspen, 1998).

3. This "way out," the focus on systems, is exactly equivalent to the "way out" of the cost quality tension that was "solved" in manufacturing industries by the philosophy associated with Total Quality Management which stressed process control. See W.E. Deming, "Improvement of Quality and Productivity through Action by Management," *National Productivity Review* 1, no. 1 (Winter 1981-1982): 12-22. For an excellent critique, see R.W. Grant, R. Shani, and R. Krishnan, "TQM's Challenge to Management Theory and Practice," *Sloan Management Review* 35, no. 2 (1994): 25-35.

4. A.E. Mills and E. M. Spencer, "Evidence-Based Medicine: Why Clinical Ethicists Should be Concerned," *HEC Forum* 15, no. 3 (Fall 2003): 231-44. Also see P. Plsek, "Redesigning Health Care with Insights from the Science of Complex Adaptive Systems," in *Crossing The Quality Chasm: A New Health System for the 21st Century* (Washington D.C.: National Academy Press; 2001).

5. For a description of how culture and values are affected by process control, see J. Detert, R.G. Schroeder, and J.J. Mauriel, "A Framework for Linking Culture and Improvement Initiatives in Organizations," *Academy of Management Review* 25, no. 4 (October 2000): 850-63.

6. A.C. Enthoven and L.A.Tollen, "Competition in Health Care: It takes Systems to Pursue Quality and Efficiency," *Health Affairs,* September 2005, *http://content.healthaffairs.org/cgi/content/abstract/hlthaff.w5.420.*

7. B. Vastag, "Physician Dissatisfaction Growing (Health Agencies Update)," *Journal of the American Medical Association* 286,

no. 7 (15 August 2001): 781.

8. S.M. Dy, H.R. Rubin, and H.P. Lehmann, "Why do patients and families request transfers to tertiary care? A qualitative study," *Social Science & Medicine* 61, no. 8 (October 2005): 1846-53.

9. R.S. Kaplan and D.P. Norton, *The Balanced Scorecard: Translating Strategy into Action* (Boston, Mass.: Harvard Business School Press, 1996).

10. B. Victor and J. Cullen, "The Organizational Bases of Ethical Work Climates," *Administrative Science Quarterly* 33 (1988) 101-25.

11. E.M. Spencer et al., *Organization Ethics in Healthcare* (New York City, New York: Oxford University Press, 2000).

12. Change, and, in particular, positive change, requires certain conditions for success that are sometimes difficult to arrange in any organization, let alone complex pluralistic organizations, and all too often deliberate strategic change fails. See M. Beer and N. Nohria, "Cracking the code of change," *Harvard Business Review*, 78, no 3. (2000): 133-141.

13. See the AHA website, *http://www.aha.org/aha/annual_meeting/content/05_reformhealthcareliab.pdf.*

14. "President Pleased by House Passage of Medical Liability Reform," *America's Intelligence Wire*, 28 July 2005.

15. "Hospitals Praise Governor's Signing of Comprehensive Medical Liability Reform Legislation," *PR Newswire,* 25 August 2005.

16. Plsek, see note 9 above.

17. M.R. Chassin, R.W. Galvin, and the National Table on Health Care Quality, "The Urgent Need to Improve Health Care Quality," *Journal of American Medical Association* 280, no. 11 (1998): 1000-5.

18. For instance, the Ethical Force program is designed to bring together multiple stakeholders to establish core healthcare ethics values that apply throughout all healthcare organizations and across the healthcare system. See *www.EthicalForce.org.*

19. P. Werhave et al., *Organizational Ethics in Healthcare: Toward a Model for Ethical Decision Making by Provider Organizations*, a report by the American Medical Association Institute of Ethics National Working Group (Chicago, Ill.: AMA, 2001).

20. S. Kalvemark et al., "Living with conflicts-ethical dilemmas and moral distress in the health care system," *Social Science & Medicine* 58, no. 6 (March 2004): 1075-84. See also A.

Jameton, *Nursing Practice: The Ethical Issues* (Englewood Cliffs, N.J.: Prentice Hall, 1984).

Appendix:
The ACGME Outcome Project General Competencies

At its February 1999 meeting, the ACGME endorsed general competencies for residents in the areas of:

- patient care,
- medical knowledge,
- practice-based learning and improvement, and
- interpersonal and communication skills,
- professionalism,
- systems-based practice.

Identification of general competencies is the first step in a long-term effort designed to emphasize educational outcome assessment in residency programs and in the accreditation process. During the next several years, the ACGME's Residency Review and Institutional Review Committees will incorporate the general competencies into their Requirements. The following statements will be used as a basis for future Requirements language. If you have any questions, comments and other requests for assistance, please address them to *outcomes@acgme.org*.

ACGME GENERAL COMPETENCIES Vers. 1.3 (9.28.99)

The residency program must require its residents to develop the competencies in the 6 areas below to the level expected of a new practitioner. Toward this end, programs must define the specific knowledge, skills, and attitudes required and provide educational experiences as needed in order for their residents to demonstrate the competencies.

PATIENT CARE

Residents must be able to provide patient care that is compassionate, appropriate, and effective for the treatment of health problems and the promotion of health. Residents are expected to:

- communicate effectively and demonstrate caring and respectful behaviors when interacting with patients and their families
- gather essential and accurate information about their patients
- make informed decisions about diagnostic and therapeutic interventions based on patient information and preferences, up-to-date scientific evidence, and clinical judgment
- develop and carry out patient management plans
- counsel and educate patients and their families
- use information technology to support patient care decisions and patient education
- perform competently all medical and invasive procedures considered essential for the area of practice
- provide health care services aimed at preventing health problems or maintaining health
- work with health care professionals, including those from other disciplines, to provide patient-focused care

MEDICAL KNOWLEDGE

Residents must demonstrate knowledge about established and evolving biomedical, clinical, and cognate (e.g. epidemiological and social-behavioral) sciences and the application of this knowledge to patient care. Residents are expected to:

- demonstrate an investigatory and analytic thinking approach to clinical situations
- know and apply the basic and clinically supportive sciences which are appropriate to their discipline

PRACTICE-BASED LEARNING AND IMPROVEMENT

Residents must be able to investigate and evaluate their patient care practices, appraise and assimilate scientific evidence, and improve their patient care practices. Residents are expected to:

- analyze practice experience and perform practice-based improvement activities using a systematic methodology
- locate, appraise, and assimilate evidence from scientific studies related to their patients' health problems
- obtain and use information about their own population of patients and the larger population from which their patients are drawn
- apply knowledge of study designs and statistical methods to the appraisal of clinical studies and other information on diagnostic and therapeutic effectiveness
- use information technology to manage information, access on-line medical information; and support their own education
- facilitate the learning of students and other health care professionals

INTERPERSONAL AND COMMUNICATION SKILLS

Residents must be able to demonstrate interpersonal and communication skills that result in effective information exchange and teaming with patients, their patients families, and professional associates. Residents are expected to:

- create and sustain a therapeutic and ethically sound relationship with patients
- use effective listening skills and elicit and provide information using effective nonverbal, explanatory, questioning, and writing skills
- work effectively with others as a member or leader of a health care team or other professional group

PROFESSIONALISM

Residents must demonstrate a commitment to carrying out professional responsibilities, adherence to ethical principles, and sensitivity to a diverse patient population. Residents are expected to:

- demonstrate respect, compassion, and integrity; a responsiveness to the needs of patients and society that supercedes self-interest; accountability to patients, society, and the profession; and a commitment to excellence and on-going professional development
- demonstrate a commitment to ethical principles pertaining to provision or withholding of clinical care, confidentiality of patient information, informed consent, and business practices
- demonstrate sensitivity and responsiveness to patients' culture, age, gender, and disabilities

SYSTEMS-BASED PRACTICE

Residents must demonstrate an awareness of and responsiveness to the larger context and system of health care and the ability to effectively call on system resources to provide care that is of optimal value. Residents are expected to:

- understand how their patient care and other professional practices affect other health care professionals, the health care organization, and the larger society and how these elements of the system affect their own practice
- know how types of medical practice and delivery systems differ from one another, including methods of controlling health care costs and allocating resources
- practice cost-effective health care and resource allocation that does not compromise quality of care
- advocate for quality patient care and assist patients in dealing with system complexities
- know how to partner with health care managers and health care providers to assess, coordinate, and improve health care and know how these activities can affect system performance

©2005 Accreditation Council of Graduate Medical Education, used with permission, all rights reserved.
http://www.acgme.org/outcome/comp/compFull.asp

Contributors

Kirsten Alcorn, MD, is Medical Director of Transfusion Services and Medical Director of Microbiology Laboratories at Washington Hospital Center in Washington, D.C., a part of MedStar Health.

Daniel M. Becker, MD, MPH, MFA, is a Professor of Medicine and Public Health Sciences and is the Director of the Center for Humanism in Medicine at the University of Virginia in Charlottesville.

Rebecca Bigoney, MD, is a Board Certified Internist who serves as a Collaborating Physician and the Director of Ethics Services at Mary Washington Hospital in Fredericksburg, Virginia.

Phil Buescher, MD, is Chief of Critical Care Medicine at Union Memorial Hospital in Baltimore, Maryland, a part of MedStar Health.

Donna T. Chen, MD, MPH, is an Assistant Professor of Public Health Sciences, Psychiatric Medicine, and Biomedical Ethics and Coordinator of Professionalism Education for the Center for Biomedical Ethics at the University of Virginia in Charlottesville.

Paul A. Clark, MPA, is Senior Knowledge Manager in the Department of Research, Service, and Strategy at Press, Ganey Associates in South Bend, Indiana.

Walter S. Davis, MD, is an Assistant Professor of Rehabilitation Medicine and Director of Education for the Center for Biomedical Ethics at the University of Virginia in Charlottesville.

Evan G. DeRenzo, PhD, is a Bioethicist in the Center for Ethics at the Washington Hospital Center in Washington, D.C., a part of MedStar Health.

Matthew J. Goodman, MD, is Associate Professor of Clinical Internal Medicine at the University of Virginia in Charlottesville.

Lisa H. Newton, PhD, is Director of the Applied Ethics Program in the College of Arts and Sciences at Fairfield University in Fairfield, Connecticut.

Natalie B. May, PhD, is an Assistant Professor and Director of Research for the Division of General Medicine, Geriatrics and Palliative Care at the University of Virginia Health Sciences Center in Charlottesville.

Ann E. Mills, Msc (Econ), MBA, is an Assistant Professor in the Center for Biomedical Ethics at the University of Virginia in Charlottesville.

David T. Ozar, PhD, is the Director at the Center for Ethics and Social Justice and is Professor of Philosophy at Loyola University of Chicago.

Mary V. Rorty, PhD, is a Clinical Associate Professor at the Stanford Center for Biomedical Ethics in Stanford, California.

Joel M. Schectman, MD, MPH, is an Associate Professor of Medicine at the University of Virginia Health System in Charlottesville.

Edward M. Spencer, MD, is semiretired; he continues as Director of Developing Healthcare Ethics Programs (DHEP) at the University of Virginia Center for Biomedical Ethics in Charlottesville, and is a consultant to a number of healthcare organizations.

John D. Voss, MD, is Associate Professor of Clinical Internal Medicine in the Division of General Medicine of the Department of Internal Medicine at the University of Virginia in Charlottesville.

Contributors

Patricia H. Werhane, PhD, has a joint appointment as Wicklander Chair of Business Ethics and Director of the Institute for Business and Professional Ethics at DePaul University in Chicago and as Ruffin Professor of Business Ethics and Senior Fellow of the Olsson Center for Applied Ethics, Darden Graduate School of Business Administration, University of Virginia, Charlottesville.

Matthew K. Wynia, MD, MPH, is Director of the Institute for Ethics at the American Medical Association.

Index

academic medical centers, 50, 51
accountability relationships, 8
Allegheny Health, Education and Research Foundation, 107
American Medical Association, 4, 75
Code of Medical Ethics, 4, 6
Anglo-American Common Law, 69
Aristotle, 135
Association of American Medical Colleges, 51

Balanced Scorecard, xiv, xv, 26-9, 44-6
    measurement, 47-8, 49-50
    values, 4-49
Baptist Health Care Corporation, 54-5
beneficence, 156
blood tests, 240-1
business practices, 7, 11

design characteristics, 102, 105
    ethical principles, 105
    flexibility, 111-3
    goals, 105
    outcomes, 107
    professionalism, 113-4
    rigidity, 111-113
    source, 110

California insurers, 57
Centers for Medicare and Medicaid Services, 57-58
Clinical Health Economics System Simulation (CHESS), 86-8
cases, 90

Clinton Plan, 73-74
conflict
    cost and quality, 109
    of commitment, 116
    of interest, 115-116
conflicting obligations system, 11
consumer, 8, 79
continuous improvement, 240
cost savings, 254
Crossing the Quality Chasm, ix, xviii
customer, 79

de-selection, 76
Dreyfus model, 187-8
Duke University Hospital System, 52-4

ethical climate, xi
    systems-informed professionalism, 30-32
evidence-based medicine, 4

fiduciary obligation, 69-71
    managers, 72
free market commitment, 70-71

General Competencies (ACGME), vii-viii, 265-8
GERD scenario, 86
Golden Mean, 239-40
Good Physician, The 153

greening the environment, 243

Healer's Art, The 160
Health Insurance Portability and
    Accountability Act of 1996, 142
healthcare
    costs, 80
    dollar, 79
hemotocrit trigger, 241
Hippocratic Oath, 68
hospice
    care, 157
    model, 157

iatrogenic anemia, 241
informed consent, 143
Institute of Medicine, ix, 4, 128, 131
    Crossing the Quality Chasm, 11
insurance companies, 76

Joint Commission on Accreditation for
    Healthcare Organizations, x, 144

leadership, xix

managed-care organization, 75
management of blood waste, 242
mental models, 24-6
mindfulness, xvii-xvii, 158-60, 187
minimal-threshold model, 229
moral
    courage, 135-6
    development, 212
    distress, 261
    imagination, 186-7
    reasoning, 185
morally safe environment, xvii, 131, 132,
    135, 138
Myriad Genetics, 107-8

narrative medicine, 161
National Oceanic and Atmospheric
    Agency, 81

needlestick injury, 241-2

organizational ethics, x-xi
    leaders, 221
    programs, 43-44, 46-47, 260-261
    reflection, 222
    rounds, 218
    systems-informed professionalism,
        257

organizations
    moral actors, 217
Outcome Project, vii
outcome-based curriculum, 211
outcomes movement, 229

palliative care, 162
participatory learning, 86
patient
    adversarial, 236-7
    costs, 93
    sympathetic, 235-6
pay-for-performance, 57
physician
    caring, 15
    character, 10
    character traits, 14
    duty, 3
    ideal behavior, 6
    moral perspective, 3-4
    outlier, 76
    patient obligation, 70
    traditional perspective, 255-6
practical health economics, 83
President's Advisory Commission on
    Consumer Protection and
    Quality, 131
principal/agent, 71
professional ethics
    professional commitment of the
        physician, 68-9
professionalism, 253
    medical ethics, 5
    traditional ideas, 5

Index

quality
    circles, 200
    committees, 199
    plan, 199

rankism, 134
reflective practice, 158
regulation, 140-2
resident training programs, 126
Robert Wood Johnson University
    Hospitals, 55-5
root cause analysis, 199-200

simulation, 86
Skinnerian theory, 135
societal
    costs, 93
stakeholder
    conflicting obligations to, 9
    role, 9
stakeholder theory, 8
supply-demand asymmetry, 8
system
    complex adaptive, 12
    core elements, 13
    ethic, 118-119
systems, xii, 23-4, 28-9, 254-5
    adaptive, ix, 24
    complex adaptive, 128-9
    degress of flexibility, 23-4
    human, 26, 8
    informed mental model, 26-29
    informed perspective, xiv, 256
    informed perspective and ACGME
        competencies, 40
    informed professionalism, xiv-xv,
        29-30, 32-35, 182, 184-185,
        256-257
        a representation of, 34
        ACGME competencies
            and, 37-9
        benefits of, 201-3
    perspective, xviii, 256

thinking, 125-6
values, 24, 255

trilemma, 74-75

unequal distribution of power, 126

University of California, 160
University of Virginia, 160

Zeno's paradox, 155

Printed in the United States
40382LVS00005B/145-165